OXFORD MEDICAL PUBLICATIONS

DISTRIBUTING HEALTH CARE

Distributing health care: Economics and ethical issues

Paul Dolan
Sheffield Health Economics Group
University of Sheffield
UK

Jan Abel Olsen
Institute of Community Medicine
University of Tromsø
Norway

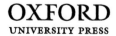

OXFORD
UNIVERSITY PRESS

OXFORD

UNIVERSITY PRESS

Great Clarendon Street, Oxford OX2 6DP

Oxford University Press is a department of the University of Oxford.
It furthers the University's objective of excellence in research, scholarship,
and education by publishing worldwide in

Oxford New York

Auckland Cape Town Dar es Salaam Hong Kong Karachi Kuala Lumpur
Madrid Melbourne Mexico City Nairobi New Delhi Shanghai Taipei Toronto

With offices in

Argentina Austria Brazil Chile Czech Republic France Greece
Guatemala Hungary Italy Japan South Korea Poland Portugal
Singapore Switzerland Thailand Turkey Ukraine Vietnam

Oxford is a registered trade mark of Oxford University Press
in the UK and in certain other countries

Published in the United States
by Oxford University Press Inc., New York

© Oxford University Press, 2002

British Library Cataloguing in Publication Data

Data available

Library of Congress Cataloging in Publication Data

Data available

ISBN 0-19-263253-1

Printed in Great Britain
on acid-free paper by
Biddles Ltd., King's Lynn, Norfolk

Preface

Health care is a unique economic commodity. In general, people do not know if and when they will need it and they do not know what types of health care they might need. They also have very little information about the impact of health care on their health. Crucially, their use of health care might impact upon other people's health and well-being. These facts make health care different from most other goods and services that are analysed in standard economic approaches. Furthermore, in most high-income countries, health care is publicly financed, and many of these countries have policy objectives that state that health care should be distributed according to some notion of need rather than according to how much consumers are willing to pay for it. All of this makes health care so interesting to us as economists and has provided the motivation for this book.

In particular, we have been motivated to write a book that is concerned with the value judgements associated with distributing health care. Our aim is to set out some of the key economic and ethical issues that are involved in distributing health care. As such, our focus follows from the desire to provide a theoretical background for analysing some of the major challenges facing health-policy makers. Indeed, we hope to show that some issues that are sometimes discussed by economists in technical language are more about policy objectives, and thus reflect normative assumptions upon which economic analyses are based.

The book is compact and has a focus on how health care should be distributed in publicly funded health care systems. It should not, therefore, be seen as a 'stand alone' textbook in health economics, but rather as a companion to other texts. We certainly acknowledge that this book does not provide a 'just coverage', in that we do not cover the topics that health economists have been writing about in proportion to the amount written on those topics. Part of this inevitably stems from our chosen walk through the topics, something that may have the unintended side-effect of stepping on the toes of some of our peers by not giving them sufficient credit. We hereby apologize, but writing a textbook that would please all of our academic colleagues is impossible—we have found it hard enough to please ourselves!

We therefore acknowledge that there are some loose ends, and there will inevitably be those who think that we should have dealt with some issues in more detail. But, as the Norwegian Nobel Laureate in Economics, Trygve Haavelmo, is said to have commented 'a good textbook should contain some weaknesses for the teacher to spot, so that he can impress his students'. With this in mind, we hope that teachers (and reviewers) will find things that they can 'score points' on! More importantly, we hope that students will gain some understanding—and enjoyment—from reading it. If they start to reflect upon and deliberate about the issues, then fine. And, if they agree with our views, then even better.

Our intention has been to make the book accessible to a wide audience of economists and non-economists. We have therefore avoided using mathematical notation so far as possible and have used diagrams only where they aid exposition. This book is truly a joint effort. We hope that this comes across in the style of the book, where we have tried to make the whole thing a seamless and coherent walk through the issues. In the economists' tradition, the two authors are listed alphabetically.

Paul Dolan,
Sheffield Health Economics Group,
University of Sheffield, UK

Jan Abel Olsen,
Institute of Community Medicine,
University of Tromsø, Norway

Acknowledgements

There are two people who in their own ways have greatly influenced our views about health economics—Bob Evans and Alan Williams. To the extent that we have professional heroes, these are the two. The *Health Economics Research Programme* at the university of Oslo (HERO) is a somewhat different hero to us—a financial one. However, this is not to forget the non-pecuniary aspects in terms of its great professional environment and friendly atmosphere. Due to us both having part-time positions in Oslo, we have been able to meet regularly in a location somewhere between Sheffield and Tromsø. Therefore, this book can justifiably be considered as one output from the HERO programme.

We would like to thank Bob Evans, Gavin Mooney, Erik Nord, Jeff Richardson, and Alan Williams for their comments on particular chapters. We are indebted to Aki Tsuchiya who acted as a kind of proofreader and who pointed out some important factual errors and omissions. The usual disclaimers apply. Happy reading!

Paul Dolan and Jan Abel Olsen
April 2002

Contents

1

Health care and health

This chapter considers what is meant by health care and health. It looks at what health care does for people, and at what the determinants of ill health are. The chapter is primarily an analytical one but it also highlights some stark inequalities in health care expenditure and health.

1.1 What is health care?

What do we mean by health care? What makes some types of resource use and some activities eligible to be termed 'health care' and others not? Answering these questions seems a sensible place to start given the title of the book. Health care is about cure, care, and prevention. Health care refers to those resources society uses in an attempt to cure them or to care for people in ill health. In addition to curing and caring for people who have already become ill, health care includes *some* of those activities that seek to prevent people becoming ill in the first place.

Cure is concerned with *improvements in health*. When a person's life is in danger, or when they suffer from an illness, a 'cure' might (1) fully restore that patient's health (for example, rescue operations); (2) improve their health, though not completely (for example, cataract operations); or (3) limit the extent to which their health deteriorates (for example, pain relief for the terminally ill). While this latter situation might not correspond with the everyday connotation of the word 'cure', it is still motivated by improving health compared to what might otherwise be the case. Care is not directly concerned with improving health; rather it seeks *to provide dignity* for sick people.

Prevention includes those resources whose main purpose is *to reduce the probability of illness or premature death*. In principle, prevention includes any intervention that seeks to reduce these risks; for example, traffic, work, and environmental safety. As such, there are many ways in which illness and premature death can be prevented, and often these lie outside of our usual conceptions of health care. One pragmatic way to separate out 'preventive health care' from other preventive interventions is to say that for prevention to be termed health care, health professionals must be involved in its provision. An even more pragmatic approach would be to say that health care is whatever a national accounting system (for example, the Organisation for Economic Co-operation and Development (OECD) system of classifying health care expenditures) defines it to be.

The three types of health care identified above differ in at least three important respects. First, they differ in their *primary purpose*. Cure and prevention primarily seek to improve health; that is, to produce health outcomes. Caring, on the other hand, has a qualitatively different purpose. The interaction between a carer and a patient is not justified by its outcomes, but by such process-related concepts as dignity, respect, autonomy, empathy, and sympathy. The economic evaluation of health care interventions has traditionally focused on the measurement of health outcomes and has largely ignored the less tangible, and consequently harder to measure, processes of care. Nonetheless, it is important to try to measure the 'goodness' from the various types of care because not all types of care are equally good.

Second, the types of health care differ according to the *availability of alternatives* to health care. There are clearly alternative measures to preventive health care. For example, in the case of anti-hypertensive drugs, there are alternative 'non-pharmacological' interventions such as reduced salt intake or physical exercise. If avoided deaths are 'produced' by prevention, then safety interventions might be better than health care at producing them. There are also substitutes for formal health care through the informal sector. Rather than being institutionalized, sick people could receive care from family members, friends, or charities. In the case of cure, however, there are very few—if any—substitutes. For most illnesses, most of us would prefer to see a health professional rather than anyone else. The extent to which alternatives to health care exist is crucial in the context of a discussion about the public provision of health care. In general, the fewer alternatives to health care that exist, the stronger the argument for public subsidisation. This is an issue we will return to later in the book.

Finally, the types of health care differ according to their *time horizon*. Whilst both cure and care deal with the present, prevention in concerned with the future. The closer in time the relationship between the intervention and its consequent 'goodness', the more 'heroic' becomes the intervention, and the more morally obliged society becomes to make health care available. As a result, there is an ethical difference between health care that saves the life of a known individual (for example, by mountain rescues) and health care that results in the saving of an unknown (statistical) life in the future (for example, by road safety).

1.2 **What is health?**

Much of the discussion so far, particularly with respect to cure and pre-vention, has focused on health care *in relation to health*. So, what is 'health' then? Defining health is even more problematic, and certainly more con-troversial, than seeking to define health care. We can think of a continuum of definitions ranging from the very narrow to the very broad. At one extreme lies a narrow medico-technical definition, where health refers to the degree of bodily functioning that is observable to an external expert and measurable on medical instruments. At the other extreme lies the famous World Health Organization (WHO) definition of health as 'a state of complete physical, mental, and social well-being' not 'merely the absence of disease and infirmity'.

Such an all-encompassing definition of health would imply that every-thing becomes health care, simply because all commodities affect 'physical, mental, and social well-being'. For the purposes of distributing health care, a narrower conception of health is required. A pragmatic approach to finding a meaningful definition of health would be to look at how health is defined within the *descriptive systems* that are currently being used to meas-ure health in clinical trials and evaluative studies. Interestingly, many of these descriptive systems refer to the concept of *health-related quality of life*, implying something that is broader than the medico-technical defini-tion of health but narrower than the WHO definition. But, of course, this still raises questions about what health means in 'health-related'.

The different descriptive systems define health in different ways, largely because they are designed for different purposes. Condition-specific instru-ments are designed to measure health within a particular condition or dis-ease group. Generic instruments have been developed to measure and compare health status across a range of different dimensions, although the dimensions often cannot be combined to form an overall single value for a composite health state because the number of dimensions and levels within dimensions is very large. There now exist some descriptive systems that do allow values to be attached to overall health status and, because these are suitable for use in informing resource allocation decisions across a range of diverse interventions, they will be the focus of attention here. Table 1.1 lists these descriptive systems together with the dimensions of health contained within them (see Brazier *et al.* 1999 and Richardson 2001). The systems differ enormously in the dimensions that they include and also markedly in terms of where they are located on the 'narrow' to 'broad' spectrum. The Health Utilities Index: Version 3 (HUI-III), for example,

Table 1.1 The different descriptive systems that generate single index values for health

Descriptive system	Dimensions	Levels	Health states
Rosser	Disability Distress	8 4	29
EQ-5D (formerly EuroQol)	Mobility, self-care, usual activities, pain/discomfort, anxiety/depression	3	243
Quality of well-being (QWB)	Mobility, physical activity, social functioning 27 symptoms/problems	3 2	1170
SF-6D (derived from SF-36)	Physical functioning, role limitations, social functioning, pain, mental health, vitality	4–6	18 000
Health Utilities Index: Version 2 (HUI-II)	Sensory, mobility, emotion cognitive, self-care, pain, fertility		24 000
Health Utilities Index: Version 3 (HUI-III)	Vision, hearing, speech, ambulation, dexterity, emotion, cognition, pain		972 000
AQoL (assessment of quality of life; or Australian QoL)	Illness, independent living, social relationships, physical senses, psychological well-being—each consists of three sub-dimensions		16 800 000

adopts a rather narrow 'within-the-skin' conception of health, whilst dimensions such as 'usual activities' put the EQ-5D (formerly EuroQol) more towards the other end of the spectrum.

Even at this pragmatic level, then, there are enormous differences in how health is defined. However, all the descriptive systems in Table 1.1 define health as being something narrower than general well-being but much wider than the presence or absence of a medical condition. This general definition of health is all that is required for the purposes of this book.

The dimensions included in these descriptive systems refer to attributes of health *states* only. As such, they all refer to the 'quality' side of health, as opposed to the 'quantity' side that takes account of *duration*. Any meaningful metric of health would clearly have to include both quality and quantity. Furthermore, when judgements are made on the *expected* gains from an intervention, the probability of successful outcomes is crucial; the higher the success rate, the better. And, lastly, at the population level, the more *people* that receive individual health gains, the higher the total health gain to society. Thus, the simplest way to value health gains would be to calculate the product of (1) health state improvements, (2) duration, (3) probability, and (4) the number of people benefiting. Calculating health gain in this or other more complicated ways is perhaps the most crucial part of the economic evaluation of health care interventions, and it is something we will return to in later chapters.

1.3 **What does health care—and health— do for people?**

The reasons why people consume health care are very different from why they consume other goods and services. In general, consumers demand goods because of the pleasure (or avoided pain) these goods are expected to yield. In the language of economists and philosophers, consumers derive *utility* from the consumption of most goods and services. In more everyday language, we get satisfaction from consuming goods—otherwise we would not have chosen to spend money on them.

The reason why patients consume health care, however, is *not* because health care gives satisfaction *per se*, but rather because of the positive effect it has on health. Thus, the demand for health care is *derived* from the demand for health. In the words of Evans and Wolfson (1980), 'health care *per se* is in general a dis-good, except in so far that it contributes to health (...). People 'consume' health care for its expected effects on health; absent these, and they would prefer not to use it'. Hence, in order for people to be willing to consume health care, the benefits in terms of expected improvements in health must more than outweigh the disutility from the consumption of health care.

So, what good does good health do then? First and foremost, good health has intrinsic value in its own right. There is a direct effect of improved health on the individual's utility. Beyond this direct effect, there are two important positive 'side-effects' of improved health. First, healthy people are able to earn more and, second, healthy people are better able to satisfy their social needs. These relationships are shown in Fig. 1.1. Health care (*HC*) and wealth (*W*) are measurable in physical or monetary terms. Social relations (*SR*) can be measured in terms of number of friends and family members, as well as the frequency of contacts with them, but this says nothing, of course, about the quality of these contacts. Health (*H*) can be

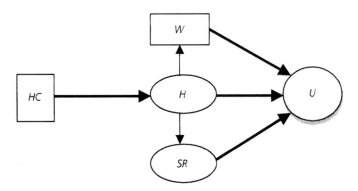

Fig. 1.1 The instrumental nature of health care—and of health. *HC*, health care; *H*, health; *W*, wealth; *SR*, social relations; *U*, utility.

measured by the various descriptive systems referred to above. Utility (*U*)—measured in units of satisfaction, which economists refer to as utils—is the hardest parameter in Fig. 1.1 to measure.

Consider first the right-hand side of the figure. Utility is what an individual would like to have the most of in life. To the left of utility are the three main 'goodies' in life which yield utility; namely, wealth, health, and social relations. Since more utility is preferred to less, more wealth, health, and social relations are also preferred to less. The popular phrase that 'it is better to be rich and healthy than poor and sick' may suggest that only wealth and health matter, but human beings are social animals, and the more social relations you have, the better you feel. Of course, there may come a point when you have too much of a good thing—you become satiated—but most of us would prefer to be rich and healthy than poor and sick. And most of us would prefer to have many friends rather than few.

In general, we can make trade-offs between the 'goodies' in life. For example, improved health can compensate for reduced wealth and, whilst 'money can't buy me love', pleasant social relations are also some compensation for reduced wealth. Of course, the precise trade-offs we make will depend on many things, some of which may be determined for us (by our backgrounds and life experiences, for example) whilst others are more directly under our control. These issues will be returned to throughout the book.

Figure 1.1 shows the crucial roles that both health care and health play in life. Beyond the direct bold arrow from health to utility, there are somewhat thinner arrows from health to wealth, and from health to social relations. Of course, the interrelations between health, wealth, and social relations are more complex than the figure indicates. For example, it has been shown that good social relations have positive health effects, and that the social position associated with high income may also yield positive health effects. For simplicity, however, such effects are not included in this figure.

We have already said that, when in need of cure, there are few—if any— substitutes to health care. Hence, access to health care is an important determinant of an individual's utility. The figure also serves to highlight the important distinction between the sphere of interest of health profession- als compared to individual patients. The sphere of health professionals is— and should be—restricted to the arrow from health care to health. They are trained to have information on the expected health effects from various types of health care. Based on this information, then, it is the sphere of the patient to judge just how important a given health improvement is for their utility—provided, of course, that they have sufficient mental capabilities to do so.

1.4 The determinants of (ill) health

The crucial public health question, 'Why are some people healthy and others not?' is discussed in a book with the same title by Evans *et al.* (1994). They consider there to be three major determinants of (ill) health in a pop- ulation: (1) *genetics*, which explains inherited diseases through natural variations in human biology; (2) *the environment*, including physical factors like working conditions and pollution and social factors like cul- tural norms and position in the social hierarchy; and (3) (health-related) *lifestyle*, that at the population level can be explained largely by cultural and social norms.

The three determinants differ in the extent to which individuals can exer- cise discretion and control over them. Genetic endowments are something which most of us take as given, no matter how hard we might fight against them. The physical and social environment is fairly given, particularly for children who have very little say over the environment they are brought up in. If they were to have a say, we might have very different social arrange- ments and very different views about what constitutes social injustice. As we get older, we come to have more freedom in choosing the environment but we are never completely without constraints.

Lifestyle is the determinant of ill health over which we have most discre- tion but precisely how much of observed behaviour reflects genuine choice and how much is due to factors outside the individual's control is a very contentious issue. Rather than consider lifestyle to be entirely within an individual's control or to be entirely determined by genetic and environmental factors, it is more helpful to consider an individual's lifestyle to be determined by a variety of factors over which they have differing *degrees of discretion*.

Figure 1.2 presents a graphical representation of the determinants of ill health. We have chosen to introduce *preferences* (rather than lifestyle) as an independent variable. This variable is to reflect genuine differences in the choices that people make. Note here that a particular preference is not unhealthy *per se*. It is when a preference is being *revealed through behaviour* that it may become unhealthy. An individual's lifestyle, then, depends upon a combination of their *responses* to the environment and their *choices* determined by their freely expressed preferences. Of course, there are moral and ideological disagreements as to which actions a person should be held responsible for, but we will not concern ourselves with this here. In reality, of course, genetics, environment, and preferences are related to one another, but for ease of exposition the possible arrows between them are not shown here. Among these determinants, the first two—at least in principle—are observable, whilst preferences are not.

Our emphasis on health-related lifestyle within this map of causation is justified on the grounds that this variable is often associated with

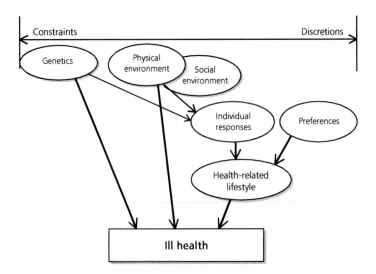

Fig. 1.2 The determinants of ill health.

self-inflicted diseases, for which, some would argue, individuals should be held responsible. However, the model suggests that a 'lifestyle-disease' is not necessarily self-inflicted, rather it may be caused by a mental or biological response to the environment in which people happens to find themselves.

What implications does Fig. 1.2 have for health care interventions? Well, the rationale behind preventive health care is to prevent ill health. The map of causality illustrates the determinants that various interventions could be targeted at. For genetics, effort would perhaps be best concentrated upon future generations because there is much less that can be done for those of us around already. For the physical and social environments, a range of environmental protection and work safety measures exist, and there are a range of policies that seek to improve housing conditions and safety in the workplace.

In order to prevent ill health through changing preferences, there are various health education programmes which seek to encourage people to depart from an unhealthy norm ('kiss a non-smoker and feel the difference' is a particular favourite of ours). With preferences, interventions become ethically more controversial. If a preference is not 'irrational' (through there being no addiction and no lack of foresight about the consequences) and if there are no negative impacts on others, it seems fully justified to defend risky and unhealthy preferences. This contrasts with a view that we should all be encouraged to choose 'the healthy way'.

Figure 1.2 raises two further interesting questions. First, at what levels are there *suitable alternatives* to preventive health care? The further back we go, the more likely that social policy and work safety will bring about greater health gains than health promotion. Second, at what level of the causal chain should health interventions be implemented? It would appear that the further back in the chain we go, the more 'side-effects' there are in terms of positive lifestyle responses. Furthermore, it seems ethically less controversial to try to change the factors that shape preferences rather than trying to shape preferences themselves (but see how tricky and circular this can all become!).

1.5 The health of nations

Health care is distributed unequally. Rather unsurprisingly, there are immense global inequalities in the distribution of health care. For example, the least developed countries spend, on average, US$11 per capita on health care compared to US$1907 in high-income countries (WHO, www.who.int/whosis/). It is also the case that health care expenditure per capita increases with national income, or gross domestic product (GDP).

Moreover, it seems to increase at a higher rate; that is, the richer a country is, the higher percentage of GDP it spends on health care. As illustrations, the USA spends 14% of its GDP on health care, most other OECD countries spend somewhere between 7% and 9%. Poor countries such as the Philippines and Kenya spend 3–4%. In fact, most analyses suggest that national income is the most important determinant of expenditure on health care.

In general, the poorer a population is, the sicker they are and the shorter they live. While GDP is the most widely used indicator for 'the wealth of a nation', life expectancy and infant mortality are the most commonly used indicators for 'the health of a nation'. More recently, the WHO has started to use disability-adjusted life expectancy (DALE) in order to express mortality and morbidity in the same index. Global differences in life expectancies at birth are wide. For example, life expectancy at birth in the least developed countries is 51 years, as compared to 78 years in high-income countries. Differences in infant mortality rates across these development categories are equally as stark. There are 100 deaths before the age of one per 100 000 live births in the least developed countries as compared to six per 100 000 in high-income countries (www.who.int/whosis/).

Whilst less dramatic, there are wide variations in health within countries, even developed ones. In the UK, for example, life expectancy amongst men in the two lowest social classes is 69.7 years, which is 5.2 years less than in the two highest social classes. These facts follow from the observation of strong social class gradients in age-standardized mortality rates across almost all diseases. Small-area analyses of mortality rates in the USA have revealed remarkable differences in life expectancy at birth across geographically defined groups. For men in 1990, it showed a difference of 16.5 years (range 61–77.5).

Thus, there is a strong relationship between wealth and health both across and within countries. Income appears to affect mortality and morbidity through different *pathways*. In the poor countries of the world, there is a clear and strong relationship between GDP per capita and life expectancy, in that small increases in wealth are related to quite substantial increases in life expectancy. Those poor countries with the highest life expectancies (such as Cuba) also tend to have higher levels of literacy. When comparing the richer countries of the world, the curve showing the relationship between per-capita GDP and life expectancy is much flatter, that is, there is a weaker relationship between income and health. This suggests that there is a diminishing marginal impact of increased income levels on life expectancy. However, this contrasts with the strong relationships between income and life expectancy *within* these rich countries.

While *biological* pathways (insufficient nutrition and infectious diseases) are posited as the primary reason why people in poor countries die early the reason why poor people in rich countries die earlier than their rich counterparts might be better explained by *psychosocial* pathways. However, it is not clear whether these health differences are due to income differences as such, or people having different positions in a social hierarchy, which is associated with inequalities in income. In the former explanation, it is deprivation and financial frustrations that produce ill health. In the latter explanation, it is subordination, lack of self-control, and low self-esteem associated with being at the bottom of a social hierarchy which produce ill health.

There are also issues, which we do not have the scope to cover in this book, relating to possible reverse causalities. That is, the extent to which those in poor health are less productive and so earn less. Determining whether and how low incomes are related to poor health and whether and how poor health is related to low incomes are hard tasks indeed.

1.6 **Conclusion**

We have taken a rather pragmatic and instrumental approach to defining health care and health. Health care consists of three branches of activities—cure, care, and prevention. Whilst health care personnel normally provide cure and care, prevention may involve a range of interventions whose overriding objective is to prevent ill health and reduce the risks of dying—of which only a part is provided by the health sector. A pragmatic definition of health care, then, is whatever happens to be classified as such in a national accounting system. In this way, we avoid a controversial distinction between what might clearly be termed health care, and what might be referred to as cosmetics.

Health is defined according to whatever descriptive system is chosen to look at the changes in health associated with different interventions. Our primary concern in this book is with these *health gains* rather than with health *per se*. We are largely concerned, therefore, with the impact of health care on health.

There are many facts and figures to prove a strong correlation between wealth and health. Figures may change but patterns remain. We recommend readers tour the web and seek updated figures. Under suggested reading, we have provided some sites to start with, as well as some interesting books that discuss alternative explanations to the facts and figures.

Suggested reading

OECD Health Data, http://www1.oecd.org/els/health/

The World Bank, http://www.worldbank.org/poverty/

The World Health Chart, http://www.whc.ki.se

WHO, http://www.who.int/whosis/

Evans, R., Barer, M., and Marmor, T. (ed.) (1994) *Why are some people healthy and others not? The determinants of health of populations.* New York: Gruyter.

Leon, D. and Walt, G. (ed.) (2001) *Poverty, inequality and health.* Oxford: Oxford University Press.

Marmot, M. and R. Wilkinson (ed.) (1999) *Social determinants of health.* Oxford: Oxford University Press.

2

Economics and efficiency

This chapter has the dual purpose of introducing the 'dismal science' of economics to non-economists, and to draw trained economists' attention to those parts of their discipline that are most relevant in the context of this book. Therefore, rather than purporting to represent a complete introduction to economics, the chapter introduces concepts and basic models which are of particular relevance later in the book.

We believe that most people perceive economics to be a discipline that primarily—if not exclusively—deals with efficiency issues. If people were to understand by efficiency the same as economists do, namely, that it may also include distributive issues, their conceptions would—to a large extent—be correct. However, to most people, efficiency is often understood more narrowly as being basically synonymous with maximizing production. In this chapter, we will try to clarify this confusion by explaining the many different meanings of the concept of efficiency. Before that, our main aim with this chapter is to try—in as simplified way as possible—to explain 'the heart of economics'.

There are many versions of a definition of economics. We rather like the definition found in *The pocket economist*: 'how scarce resources are used to produce and distribute goods and services to meet human wants'. Because one of its early practitioners, Malthus, believed that scarcity was so acute as to put the world permanently on the edge of famine, economics came to be known as the 'dismal science'. Therefore, three main concepts—production, distribution and scarcity—are embodied in 'the heart of economics'.

Economists try to answer three questions simultaneously—*What* is to be produced, *how* is it to be produced, and *for whom* is it to be produced? As to the first question, most mainstream economists would say that people's preferences should determine what is to be produced, that is, 'give the people what they want'. Alternatively, some would argue that people's needs should determine what is to be produced. This distinction between 'wants' (or 'desires') and 'needs' is particularly relevant in the context of health care, and is therefore something we shall return to. How things are to be produced depends on technology, as well as the relative prices of the factors of production. Most economists would agree that a given level of a particular good or service should be produced in the cheapest way possible.

For whom, is an issue of distribution, and the answer given by conventional models is to distribute the goods according to people's willingness and ability to pay. This is how the problem of distribution is solved in model markets as well as in many real world markets. However, this distributive principle is more value laden than many economists would like to acknowledge. Interestingly, in those countries with publicly funded health care, an overriding objective is to distribute health care quite independently of people's willingness and ability to pay for such services.

When answering these fundamental questions, economics emerges as a field somewhere at the interface between engineering and ethics. Economists would ask engineers about what is technologically feasible, that is, how can we possibly produce the things that people want (or need)? And they would ask politicians about which distributive principle society wants as a basis for determining who are to have these things. Thus, when the technologies have been identified and the distributive principles have been decided, the economist springs into action.

Economic models have three types of building blocks: (1) identities, (2) technological relations, and (3) the objective function. A typical 'identity' relationship for a producer is the account balance, that is, 'money out = money in'. In other words, the revenues obtained from selling the good are equal to the costs of purchasing the input factors plus any profits. An example of a technological relation would be a production function that explains the relationship between input factors and output.

Since an optimal allocation of resources crucially depends on what we want to achieve, all economic models must also have an objective function, even if this is only stated implicitly. This objective function must also specify the appropriate distribution of resources in question. For instance, if we want to maximize health, health care would be allocated differently compared to how it would be allocated if the objective were to be doing the most good for the most severely ill.

In dealing with each of these building blocks, economic models make a number of assumptions about the way in which inputs and outputs relate to one another (see the production function below) and about how producers and consumers behave. Producers are assumed to maximize profit. In competitive markets, this behaviour is forced upon producers because they would go out of business if they did not seek to maximize profits.

Identities and technological relations are considered to be positive issues whilst stating the objective function and the distributive principles are normative issues. Positive issues deal with how things are, while normative issues deal with how things ought to be. This distinction is very important and is often strongly emphasized in economics. However, economists often have different views as to which parts of their models to label positive and which to label normative.

In the particular context of applying economic models to inform health policy, we would hold that it is for society to state the objectives and the principles under which health care should be distributed. These are therefore clearly normative issues, which might narrow the degrees of freedom that economists have when choosing which types of models to use. Beyond these explicit policy issues, there are often implicit normative issues hidden in the economic models we use. Our own—admittedly normative—view here is that analysts should be honest and explain any such distributive implications of their models. We have forced ourselves to try to do so in this book!

Our discipline is usually divided between 'macroeconomics' and 'microeconomics', as can be seen from the titles of most introductory textbooks in economics. Although the boundaries between macro- and microeconomics are often quite blurred, the majority of health economics has its theoretical basis in microeconomics.

2.1 Microeconomics—studying markets and their actors

Microeconomics focuses on the behaviour of market actors, and analyses how their behaviour influences supply and demand, and, hence, prices and quantities. Beyond this core, microeconomics includes a range of sub-disciplines, for example welfare economics and game theory.

Starting from basics, the actors in the market are usually referred to as 'producers' and 'consumers', and sometimes as firms and households, or simply sellers and buyers. Producers are assumed to be 'only in it for the money', that is, they are motivated by maximizing profits. Their behaviour is constrained by technology as well as by prevailing market prices. Under 'perfect competition' each producer is a 'price taker', that is, their quantities are so small relative to the size of the market that they do not individually influence market prices. However, under other market forms, a single producer may influence the market price, as would be the case under monopoly where there is only one producer in the market.

Consumers are assumed to be 'only in it for the pleasure', that is, they are motivated by maximizing utility. Their choices are constrained by their income and the prevailing market prices. The moves they make depend on their individual 'taste'. In the following sub-sections, we examine some important aspects of microeconomic models.

2.1.1 More in means more out—but at a diminishing rate

Production functions

A production function sets out the 'technology relationship', explaining how the amounts of input factors, such as labour and machinery, vary with the production of goods. Usually we find that production increases with more input, although it rarely increases proportionally with input. Initially, production would often increase more than the increase in input, and we have what is termed 'economies of scale'. After some level of production, this 'overproportional' increase starts to diminish to the point where there is 'constant return to scale', that is, production increases proportionally with input. After this level, there is 'underproportional' increase—production increases at a diminishing rate. The good thing, though, is that production still increases with more input. But, most good things come to an end, and there comes a point where more input does not yield more output (termed the 'satiation point'), after which more input would actually reduce the level of output. Figure 2.1 illustrates this pattern, where the horizontal axis, labelled L, is the amount of labour used, and the vertical axis, X, is the amount of goods produced.

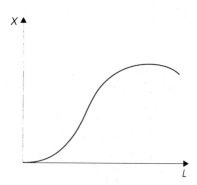

Fig. 2.1 The typical relationship between one input, L, and one output, X.

This S-shaped production function has intuitive appeal. Consider doctors as an input factor. With a given hospital equipped with various types of machinery, one doctor would spend much time running from one end of the building to the other. Employing more doctors means that less time would be wasted. When all the wasted time has been saved, more doctors may still lead to increased production, because they can specialize and help each other. The production will increase, but at a diminishing rate. Then, there comes a point, beyond which more doctors would get in each other's way, so that production will actually fall.

The central concept of productivity must not be forgotten here. This can be defined on an average or marginal basis. Average productivity is simply the total output divided by the number of units of the particular input: in the case of labour, this is X/L. Marginal productivity is the additional output which follows from employing an additional unit of the particular input: in the case of labour, this is dX/dL where d means change. The average or marginal productivity depends crucially on how much other inputs are involved. Labour productivities would normally be higher the more machinery there is behind each employee. So, as well as different paces of work, differences in labour productivity across countries may also be due to differences in how much machinery is available.

As to the optimal number of workers to employ, not much can be said on the basis of this general production function alone. The only thing we can say for sure is not to employ beyond the satiation point, at which new workers will only mess things up. The number of workers to employ will depend on the price of the input (the wage) and the price of the goods (as well as on the level and relative price of capital). The good thing about such production functions is that the relationships they are based upon can actually be measured in physical units. As such, they differ from utility functions, to which we now turn.

Utility functions

A utility function sets out the relationship between the amounts of various goods consumed and the utility that a consumer derives from them. The general relationship between the units of a particular good consumed and utility (holding other goods constant) is assumed to be somewhat simpler than with the production function above. Utility increases with more units consumed, but again at a diminishing rate. After a satiation point, the utility begins to fall (see Fig. 2.2 where the horizontal axis, labelled X, is the amount of a good consumed, and the vertical axis, U, is the utility that the consumer derives).

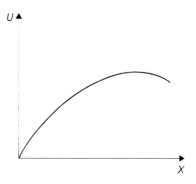

Fig. 2.2 The relationship between units consumed, X, and the utility derived, U.

We believe that most people will agree with the general shape of this utility function. For any good you consume (chocolate, say), the amount of satisfaction you get from succeeding units of that good diminishes. This is sometimes referred to as 'the law of diminishing marginal utility'. And after a certain level (again referred to as the satiation point), you realize that you wish you had not had the last unit. The average utility is simply the total amount of utility enjoyed divided by the number of units consumed to get that amount of utility (U/X). Marginal utility is then defined as the additional utility one gets from an extra unit of the particular good dU/dX.

Unfortunately, it is hard to measure utility in any meaningful unit. Whilst you might be able to attach relative utilities to additional units of a good (for example, 'the second chocolate gave half the satisfaction compared to the first one'), it is difficult—if not impossible—to express absolute levels of utility. The way in which a consumer's utility is usually measured is through their willingness to pay for the particular unit. Holding everything else constant—which from now on will be termed *ceteris paribus*—the more a consumer is willing to pay for a good, the more utility they are considered to get from that good.

But, of course, an individual's willingness to pay will be related to their income. A rich person might be willing to spend more on a chocolate than a poor person, not necessarily because she gets greater utility from the chocolate, but simply because she can afford to pay more for it. So, the way conventional economic theory measures how much utility a consumer gets is by a metric that is income dependent.

2.1.2 Substitution—'there is more than one way to skin a cat'

Substituting production factors

Most goods require the use of more than one input factor in the production process. In the following, we will stick to the conventional factors of labour and capital (or machinery):

$$X = f(L, K). \tag{2.1}$$

Suppose that a given quantity, X_0, is produced with a particular combination of labour and capital, L_0 and K_0, and that the marginal productivity of each factor is positive (that is, we are not at or beyond the satiation point). If we were to reduce labour by a certain amount ($L_1 < L_0$) while still maintaining the initial quantity, X_0, we would have to use more capital ($K_1 > K_0$). Equally, if less capital were to be used ($K_2 < K_0$), we would have to employ more labour ($L_2 > L_0$) in order to maintain X_0.

Thus, by identifying all combinations of labour and capital that produce a given quantity, an 'isoquant' (equal quantity) can be depicted. In Fig. 2.3, the horizontal axis indicates the amount of labour, L, and the vertical axis the amount of capital, K. The three combinations of labour and capital are shown as points on the isoquant that produces output X_0.

The downward slope of the isoquant shows that if we use less of one input factor, we have to compensate for this by using more of the other factor. The isoquant is convex to the origin because of diminishing marginal productivity. When we use a lot of one factor, the succeeding units of it are less productive than the preceding units. Hence, we have to use an increasing

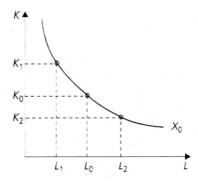

Fig. 2.3 A given quantity produced with various combinations of labour, L, and capital, K.

number of extra units in order to compensate for a reduced unit of the alternative factor. At the same time as the alternative factor is being reduced, we forego a higher and higher marginal productivity the more we reduce it.

So, why did we find it necessary to discuss isoquants? Firstly, because it is important to be reminded that there is more than one way to skin a cat, more than one way to save a life, more than one way to treat an illness and so on. Admittedly, the range of alternative options are not so many that they can be identified on a continuous smooth and elegant isoquant, but in most instances it is feasible to choose between alternative technologies—different combinations of inputs—in health care.

Secondly, isoquants help to explain two levels of efficiency. First, there is technical efficiency which means that a combination on the isoquant is chosen. This means that we do not waste input factors. If a point to the north-east of the isoquant were chosen to produce the same quantity, we would be using more input factors than necessary. It would then be possible to reduce the amount of labour or capital without reducing the quantity produced.

Which point on the isoquant should we choose? The answer is to choose the cheapest combination of inputs. This second level of efficiency is referred to as cost-efficiency. The exact point chosen on the isoquant will depend on the relative prices of the input factors. In Fig. 2.4, a budget line has been added to illustrate the relative prices of labour and capital. If wages increase, the line becomes steeper and labour is substituted with capital. Conversely, if capital costs increase, the line becomes flatter and

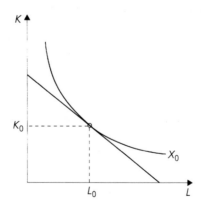

Fig. 2.4 The cost-effective combination of input factors, labour, L, and capital, K.

capital is substituted with labour. The budget line in Fig. 2.4 is tangential to the point (L_0, K_0), showing this to be the most cost-efficient combination of labour and capital.

When comparing the choice of technology between countries, we find that where labour is cheap, more of it is used relative to capital. In rich countries, on the other hand, where labour is expensive, firms tend to use relatively more capital in the production process. This is true of health care too, where poorer countries tend to spend relatively more on labour than in developed countries.

Of course, much depends on the time period over which decisions are made. In the short run, with buildings and machinery installed, it may be hard to suddenly opt for an alternative technology. Consequently, most economics textbooks assume that in the short run capital is a fixed factor of production whilst labour is a variable factor. In the long run, there is more discretion about which point on the isoquant to choose since both capital and labour are assumed to be variable. (Precisely when the short run finishes and the long run starts is rarely defined; they are simply conceptual devices.)

Substituting consumption goods

Even the saddest child can be compensated when he has to give up a toy. Give him a different toy, an ice cream or a video, and you observe a simple point: if we have to forego a unit of one good, the lost utility (or well-being or satisfaction or happiness) can be compensated by the utility obtained from more of the other good that is made available. Analogous to the fact that there is more than one way to skin a cat, there is certainly more than one way to get some satisfaction.

Consider a simplified and typical utility function, where a consumer gains utility, U, from the two goods, X and Y:

$$U = u(X, Y). \tag{2.2}$$

Imagine that a particular combination of the two goods, X_0 and Y_0, yields a given level of satisfaction, U_0. If the individual has to give up one unit of X, compensation is required in terms of more Y. The minimum compensation required in order to remain at the initial utility level is that which brings them to Y_1:

$$U_0 = u(X_0, Y_0) = u(X_1, Y_1). \tag{2.3}$$

Figure 2.5 illustrates an indifference curve that shows those combinations of two goods that yield a given level of utility for a particular consumer. You

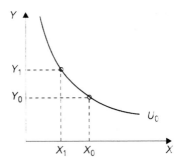

Fig. 2.5 A given utility level obtained from various combinations of two goods, X and Y.

can see that there are some similarities with isoquants that show those combinations of two inputs that yield a given output.

Like isoquants, indifference curves slope downwards from left to right—in order to remain equally happy, less Y requires more X. And like isoquants, indifference curves are convex to the origin—the reason lies in the above concept of diminishing marginal utility. The more you get of one good, the less additional utility you get from each extra unit, and so you require more of it to compensate you for the loss of the other good. At the same time, the less you get of the other good, the higher is the lost utility from each additional unit foregone, and so you require even more of the other good in compensation. The slope of the curve illustrates the consumers' marginal rate of substitution between X and Y (MRS_{XY}), that is, the number of Y required for being willing to forego one additional X.

So, what is so special about indifference curves except for their elegance? The answer is that they illustrate probably the most important attribute of consumer behaviour, namely that we make trade-offs. Such trade-offs are made not only between apples and oranges, but between fruit and chocolate, between food and wine, between cars and holidays, and between wealth (income) and health.

Unfortunately, indifference curves are not observable and cannot be measured in the same way that isoquants can. Rather, indifference curves are mental constructions—at least within the minds of economists. They crucially reflect the taste of the given consumer. Human beings are uniquely different, and consumers are sovereign in expressing their tastes. Thus, while some consumers may appear to have pretty weird preference structures, there is no 'right' or 'wrong' shape to their indifference curves.

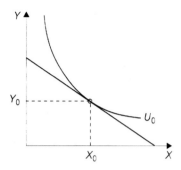

Fig. 2.6 The preferred combination of two goods, X and Y.

However, there are some restrictions that economists impose on just how weird an individual's preference function can be. One of the most important restrictions is that preferences must be transitive. This means that if you prefer A to B and B to C, then you should also prefer A to C. So, if we know you prefer hot-dogs to hamburgers and hamburgers to pizza, then we can infer that you prefer hot-dogs to pizza. If you did not, then you would be an irrational consumer.

Given all these combinations of goods that yield the same level of utility, which one would the consumer choose? The answer, analogous to that for production, is that they would choose the cheapest combination, which will be determined by the relative prices of the goods in question. In Fig. 2.6, the budget line illustrates the relative prices of X and Y. The budget line is tangential to the indifference curve at (X_0, Y_0) and here the consumer maximizes utility.

If the price of X increases (or the price of Y falls), the budget line becomes steeper and the consumer would substitute X with more of Y. If the price of X falls (or the price of Y increases), the budget line becomes flatter and the consumer would choose to consume more of X and less of Y.

2.1.3 Scarcity: a dismal reality for the dismal science

Had it not been for the constraints on input factors in Fig. 2.4, society could have moved further north-east in the output space in order to increase production. And were it not for budget constraints, most of us would fly off further north-east in the utility space to a utopian point where satiation is reached for all the goods we desire. But, unfortunately, we face scarcity of resources in the real world.

Most input factors, such as raw materials, capital, technology, skills, and labour, have limited availability. The economic problem, then, is how to allocate the available inputs across different sectors or firms that produce different goods. Consider the typical model of two input factors, labour and capital, which are available in fixed quantities, L_0 and K_0. These input factors can be used for producing either of two goods, X and Y.

If all inputs were used to produce X, there would be nothing left to produce Y, and vice versa. Imagine that we start by producing only Y. If one less unit of Y was produced, the factors required to produce this unit would be released and could be reallocated to produce as many units of X as possible. The production of Y could be reduced still further, thus transferring more and more factors to the production of X. What emerges, then, is another elegant curve: the production possibility frontier (PPF), or transformation curve, as shown in Fig. 2.7.

The reason for its downward slope is that more input factors devoted to the production of Y means fewer input factors devoted to the production of X, and so more units of Y produced means fewer units of X produced. The PPF is concave to the origin because of diminishing marginal productivities for each of the factors of production. Incremental units of labour and capital devoted to the production of Y will produce fewer additional units of Y. As inputs are taken away from the production of X, more and more units of X will have to be foregone in order to produce fewer and fewer additional units of Y.

The terms PPF and transformation curve are indicative of what the curve in Fig. 2.7 shows. They also capture concepts that lie at the heart of economics. The PPF indicates the maximum amount of one good that can be

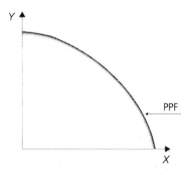

Fig. 2.7 The production possibility curve for two goods, X and Y.

produced given the amount of the other good that is produced. The collection of frontier points is referred to as being *Pareto efficient*. This means that, at any point on the frontier, it is not possible to increase the production of one good without also reducing the production of the other good. Clearly, points inside the frontier cannot be Pareto efficient. If we are inside the PPF, it would be possible to move to a point on the frontier by increasing the production of one good without reducing the production of the other.

The alternative name for the PPF—the transformation curve—literally suggests that (the production of) one good can be transformed into (the production of) the other good. This is achieved by withdrawing input factors from the production of one good and putting them into the production of the other good. Hence, the alternative to producing an extra unit of one good is what might otherwise have been produced of the other good. The slope of the transformation curve illustrates the marginal rate of transformation between X and Y (MRT_{XY}). What we forego in terms of lost production of the other good is referred to as the opportunity costs of producing an extra unit of one good. The shape of the curve in Fig. 2.7 tells us that the opportunity costs of producing incremental units of X increases, that is, more and more units of Y have to be forgone for each additional unit of X that is produced.

A frontier point is always superior to an interior point but which frontier point should we choose? The answer is that it all depends on the preferences of the consumer. If they have a strong preference for X over Y, then more of X should be produced, and vice versa. The point at which an individual consumer's indifference curve is tangential to the PPF is exactly where their utility is maximized, as shown in Fig. 2.8.

At point E, the given amounts of the factors of production have been allocated between the production of the two goods so as to reflect what people want. This unique combination of the two goods corresponds with allocative efficiency. This top-level efficiency requires that the marginal rate of transformation between X and Y (MRT_{XY}) is equal to the consumers' marginal rate of substitution between X and Y (MRS_{XY}). If unequal, it is possible to bring about a Pareto improvement. For example, if $MRT_{XY} = 2$ and $MRS_{XY} = 1$, then the economy can transform one X into two Y. Since individuals are indifferent between one X and one Y, by producing two more units of Y and one less unit of X, one individual can be made better off.

Many microeconomics textbooks include models in which two consumers trade between two different goods, whose total quantities are given

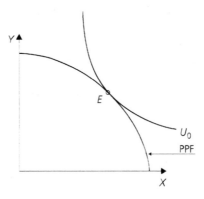

Fig. 2.8 The production possibility frontier (PPF) and utility maximization.

and whose distribution between the two consumers have been randomly determined 'like manna from heaven'. It is unlikely that the individuals' initial bundles would correspond with their respective tastes for the goods. However, by voluntarily exchanging goods with each other, an optimal distribution can be achieved. Since the exchange is voluntary, neither of them would be made worse off than initially, but their relative utility gains would depend on their relative negotiations skills. With sufficiently many different initial distributions of the two goods between the two individuals, a curve of optimal distribution can be observed to result from these exchanges.

Based on this curve, a frontier can be derived which depicts the collection of all optimal distributions of the two goods between the two individuals—the utility possibility frontier (UPF) in Fig. 2.9. The UPF shows all points where Pareto optimality exists, that is, at any point on the frontier where it is not possible for one individual to increase their utility without the other individual having to reduce theirs. Clearly, points inside the frontier cannot be Pareto optimal. The shape of the UPF will be determined by the extent to which the two individuals are able to generate utility from the goods they consume. The precise point on the UPF that is reached will depend on the initial distribution of goods between the two individuals and on their relative bargaining skills.

The frontier intersects the axes in two extreme distribution points. At U_A^{max}, A's utility is maximized by their consuming everything available of the two goods (nothing left for B). The other extreme is at U_B^{max}, where B

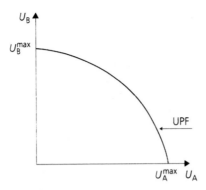

Fig. 2.9 The utility possibility frontier (UPF).

has got it all. At least two important things should be said about the UPF. First, it is based on individualistic utility functions, which means that each individual is only concerned about his own utility, something that is obtained from his own consumption of goods. Second, the UPF in itself offers no guidelines as to the ranking of preferred distributions. All points are equally 'optimal' according to the Pareto criterion, even the most extreme points. It is in Chapter 3 that we will attempt to identify ethically acceptable distributions.

2.1.4 **Supply and demand—and the magic equilibrium**

From the above models, it is implied that the more we produce of one good, the more it 'costs' in terms of foregone production of other goods. And, the more you have consumed of one good, the less you are willing to pay for it in terms of foregone consumption of other goods. In this section, we shall consider the interaction between producers and consumers in the market for one good, in isolation from the market for other goods.

When considering what determines the supply of good X, we begin by reminding ourselves about the diminishing marginal productivity of each input factor. Therefore, more input factors are needed to produce each incremental unit X. When the price of an input factor is unaffected by how much of it a producer employs, it follows that the cost of producing each additional unit will increase. Beyond this 'technical reason' for increasing marginal costs, there might be an 'input price reason' in that an input factor might become more expensive the more of it that is employed. In general, then, it seems reasonable to assume that producers are faced with increasing marginal costs.

Because each producer is assumed to try to maximize profits, they will not sell any unit of output at a loss, at least not in the long run (in the short run, he might be able to sustain losses providing these are covered by increased profits subsequently). If the market price is higher than the cost of producing the last unit, he will expand production, and hence supply increases. Conversely, if the market price is lower than the marginal costs of production, supply will be reduced. As a result, the long run supply curve is identical to the marginal cost curve. By aggregating each producer's supply curve, we have the market supply curve. And so the higher the market price, the higher the market supply.

We noted earlier that a consumer is denied reaching their satiation point by their income and the price of the good. If a consumer is willing (and able) to pay more for an additional unit of the good than its prevailing market price, then they would buy it. If their willingness to pay for the good were less than the market price, they would not buy it. The maximum amount a consumer is willing to pay for an extra unit of the good signals how much they value the benefits from that extra unit.

In general, each consumer is assumed to have a demand curve that reflects how much they value incremental units of the good. The amount that each of us demands at a given price will depend on our income and on our preferences. But it seems reasonable to assume that if the price of a good were to fall (rise), we would be more (less) inclined to buy an extra or an initial unit of the good. Analogous to the above aggregation to determine a market supply curve, when we aggregate each consumer's demand curve, we have the market demand curve. And so the lower the market price, the higher the market demand.

Figure 2.10 illustrates the typical market with an upward sloping supply curve, S, and a downward sloping demand curve, D. The horizontal axis is the quantity, Q, and the vertical axis is the price, P. The intersection between S and D determines the equilibrium price and quantity. At this point, the cost to producers of the last unit is exactly equal to the value that consumers place on this unit. For many economists, this location represents their imagination of a Nirvana!

The curves in Figure 2.10 could be relatively steep (that is, closer to being a vertical line) or relatively flat (that is, closer to being a horizontal line). The steepness of a demand (supply) curve shows the responsiveness of quantity demanded (supplied) to changes in price. A relatively steep demand

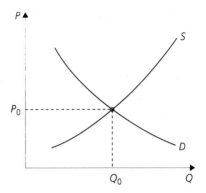

Fig. 2.10 Market equilibrium where supply, *S*, equals demand, *D*.

curve means that the quantity demanded is not very sensitive to the price of the good. A relatively flat demand curve means that the quantity demanded is sensitive to the price of the good. There are several factors that influence the steepness of the demand curve. These include (1) the availability of substitutes—where there are few close substitutes available, the demand curve will be steeper; (2) the proportion of income spent on the commodity—where the cost of the good is a small proportion of total expenditure, the demand curve will be steeper; (3) whether the good is a necessity or a luxury—if a good is considered a necessity, the demand curve will be steeper; and (4) whether the good is habit-forming—if it is, the demand curve will be steeper.

There are several factors that influence the steepness of the supply curve. These include (1) the time period—in the short run supply curves are relatively steep due to the existence of fixed factors which limit the scope for increased output, whilst in the long run supply curves are flatter because all factors are assumed to be variable; (2) factor mobility—the greater the mobility of the factors of production, the flatter the supply curve; and (3) the availability of stocks—where a product can be stored without loss of quality or undue expense, the supply curve will tend to be relatively flat.

As well as movements up and down particular demand and supply curves, we can also consider shifts in the curves. A shift in the demand curve would be caused by a change in other parameters in the demand function besides price. For example, higher incomes tend to shift the demand curve further out. The curve would also shift out when suppliers (perhaps through advertising) persuade consumers that the good is even better or even more needed than consumers had originally thought. In health economics, the concept of supplier-induced demand is illustrated by such shifts in the demand curve—here, demand is induced by doctors who recommend that patients use more health care. A shift in the supply curve is typically caused by technological changes, whereby marginal costs change, for example, technological innovation would make the supply curve shift downwards. All exogenous shifts in the demand or supply curve result in a new equilibrium for price and output.

2.2 Conclusion

The equilibrium point at which demand equals supply offers an attractive theoretical solution to 'the grand economic problem' of how much to produce in order to maximize welfare. The interaction between producers and consumers, each of them acting out of their own self-interest, brings about an optimal outcome where social welfare is maximized. The idea that an 'invisible hand' can bring about allocative efficiency has been immensely attractive to economists since Adam Smith introduced this parable more than 200 years ago.

However, like many things that look fine on paper, the 'invisible hand' is troublesome in the real world where a range of restrictive assumptions will have to be satisfied. The most important ones are that (1) suppliers and demanders are so numerous that individual actions do not impact upon the market price; (2) the good offered by each supplier is homogeneous; and (3) each consumer has full information about the good. Beyond these assumptions there are others which are of particular relevance when discussing the usefulness of 'markets' for distributing health care. These will be explained in Chapters 4 and 5. It is worth noting here, though, that the allocation that would result from a perfect market serves as a useful benchmark by which to judge other allocations by other market and non-market structures.

Suggested reading

See any introductory economics text; we recommend Part 1 of Dobson, S. and Palfreman, S. (1999) *Introduction to economics*. Oxford: Oxford University Press.
The more advanced reader (third year undergraduate level) could take a look at Part 1 of Mas-Colell, A., Whinston, M., and Green, J. (1995) *Microeconomic theory*. Oxford: Oxford University Press.

3

Justice and fairness

Justice and fairness essentially deal with two issues; whether the distribution of something is considered 'just' and 'fair', and whether the procedures that led to that distribution are considered 'just' and 'fair'. This chapter discusses the major theories of justice, with an emphasis on comparing them with each other. Given the title and focus of this book, most space will be devoted to theories of distributive justice.

The major theories of justice place different emphasis on distributive compared with procedural issues. Theories of *distributive justice* concentrate on the outcomes of a distribution whereas theories of *procedural justice* are concerned with how those outcomes came about. The arguments used by the major theories of justice to justify deviations from equality focus either on aggregate *consequences* (for example, an unequal distribution is required to increase 'the size of cake') or on the *procedures* (such as fair and democratic principles) that cause the resultant unequal distribution.

However, before meaningful comparisons between competing theories can be made, it must be recognized that the theories have very different views about which entities are to be distributed. Alternative conceptions of what is to be distributed may have very different implications for what the most efficient allocation of resources looks like. Therefore, we must first of all clarify what the 'distribuendum' is. In what follows, the entities to be distributed are divisible, so that it makes sense to have different quantities of them, and also to assume that they are preferred in larger rather than smaller amounts.

Economists have traditionally adopted the utilitarian philosophy when considering how welfare should be defined and how it should be distributed across society. Classical utilitarianism can be seen as a combination of three requirements:

(1) welfarism—the goodness of a state is a function only of the utility information regarding that state;

(2) sum-ranking—utility information can be assessed only by looking at the sum-total of utilities across individuals;

(3) consequentialism—every choice or valuation must be ultimately determined by the consequent states of affairs.

'New' welfare economics eschews cardinal utility (the idea that utility can be expressed on a numeric scale with certain properties) and interpersonal comparisons (the idea that A's utility can be compared with B's utility), and has been referred to as 'ordinal utilitarianism'. But what precisely is utility? What alternative conceptions of well-being are there? What alternatives to sum-ranking are there? And might the processes by which an outcome is achieved also matter? Each of these questions is dealt with in this chapter.

3.1 *What* is to be distributed?

3.1.1 Utility

In Chapter 2, it was shown that an efficient allocation of resources requires the *utility* possibility frontier (UPF) to be identified. Therefore, economists usually focus on individual utility. Defining an individual's welfare in terms of the utility (or happiness) they derive owes much to the work of the utilitarian philosophers, Jeremy Bentham and John Stuart Mill. The original hedonistic perspective of Bentham is based on the simple premise that people do things to attain pleasure and to avoid pain. He believed that pleasure promotion and pain avoidance could be measured cardinally as a number of *utils*, which could then be used to make interpersonal comparisons, and thus provide information regarding how much more happy one person is compared to another.

Bentham was neutral about the sources of pleasure and pain—it is for individuals to decide these things for themselves. Mill, however, distinguished between 'higher' and 'lower' pleasures, famously claiming that 'It is better to be a human being dissatisfied than a pig satisfied; better to be Socrates dissatisfied than a fool satisfied'. The view that some types of consumption patterns are more approved of than others implies that society should weight pleasures in accordance with them being of a 'higher' or a 'lower' order.

From Mill onwards, utilitarian philosophers have shown increasing interest in the *source* of an individual's utility. Although a fully informed rational person is still taken to be the best judge of their own welfare, recent models do allow for preferences to be 'laundered' in various ways. This might be to correct them for mistaken beliefs or to allow for the exclusion of certain anti-social preferences, such as envy and malice. Therefore, whilst the distribuendum in a utilitarian framework is obviously still utility, it is far from obvious *what types* of utility should be allowed to contribute towards social welfare.

All utilitarian and standard economic models do, however, rely on an individual's subjective assessment of their own utility. The crucial distributional issue is how many utils one individual is capable of generating from the consumption of an additional unit of a good as compared to how many utils another individual is capable of generating from the same unit. In viewing individuals as locations of their respective utilities, Rawls (1982) argues that utilitarianism ignores 'the separability of persons'. As such, using utility as the distribuendum can be criticised on the grounds that it treats individuals as nothing more than passive carriers of pleasure and pain.

Moreover, the *reason* why one individual may obtain more utility from a particular good consumed than another individual is not an issue: one may have different needs or one may just simply be a more effective 'pleasure-generating machine', that is, they may be easier to please. But there are circumstances (for example, when deciding whether or not to give money to a beggar) where we will make our decision based upon what we think the person 'needs' rather than on what they want. In this way, we may wish to feed a beggar, but not to finance his gambling, say.

Ignoring the source of differences in individual utility may have damaging limitations in the context of interpersonal comparisons of well-being (Sen 1987). Given that the amount of utility that an individual gets is largely determined by their experiences and expectations, it might well happen that a deprived poor person (with relatively low expectations) gets less utility from a health improvement than a richer person does. If health care were to be distributed according to the utilitarian principle, then the rich person would get the treatment. This is a solution that seems to contradict widely shared conceptions of fairness. Using Sen's terms, we might consider deprived poor people to be 'unable to manage to desire adequately'.

Another problem with measuring welfare through utility is that something valuable may be lost if it is not desired by anyone. For example, a person may not have the courage to desire freedom under an oppressive regime. The extent to which information other than that relating to individual utility is relevant to distributive judgements is one of the central issues involved in disputing utilitarianism and the Pareto principle. Sen (1987) argues that well-being may be better represented by the freedom that the person has, and not entirely by what the person achieves on the basis of that freedom. In addition, there may be social value (but not individual utility) attached to the concept of duty, or the Kantian ethic.

Such considerations take us in the direction of rights and liberties, which will be dealt with later. For now, the question that arises is 'if not utility, then what?'.

3.1.2 Primary goods

Rawls (1971) defines individual well-being in terms of an index of primary goods. These goods are (1) basic liberties, for example, freedom of thought; (2) freedom of choice of occupation; (3) powers and prerogatives of office; (4) income and wealth; and (5) social bases of self-respect. This is a rather heterogeneous list and, although Rawls saw income and wealth as acting as more easily measurable proxies for some of the other primary goods, many have criticised Rawls for having a rather vague distribuendum. Moreover, Rawls says very little about how items in the index are to be weighted and so he offers little guidance about how the primary goods are to be traded off against one another in the construction of the index.

However, Rawls does avoid some of the interpersonal comparability problems by defining an 'objective list' of primary goods. This objective list is something which society defines as being important to its *citizens*, as opposed to a welfare economic approach to subjectively valued goods within *consumers'* utility functions. Primary goods would then represent a sub-set of all possible attributes within a consumer's utility function. Having said that, whilst utility in the form of happiness may be seen as an inadequate guide to a person's well-being, Rawls asserts that it is *irrelevant* to well-being, which is a very strong claim indeed.

Interestingly, Rawls' theory applies to individual's who are 'normal, active, and fully co-operating members of society over the course of a complete life' (Rawls 1982). As noted by Daniels (1985), '*there is no distributive theory for health care because no one is sick*' [italics in original]. Is there something about Rawls' distribuendum which makes it less applicable to health care? The point made by Daniels is that while the need for Rawls' primary goods are more or less the same for everyone, there is a much more unequal distribution of the need for health care due to biological differences between people. There would then be much wider variation in the resources required to meet such unequal distributions of needs in order to compensate those who have been unfortunate to be born sick.

Rawls (1982) himself recognizes this limitation and suggests that the resources devoted to meeting the health needs of people could be decided in the light of existing social conditions. However, he argues against a cardinal and interpersonally comparable measure of health on the grounds that people in a pluralist society may have irreconcilable views about what constitutes a good life. Daniels (1985), however, has extended Rawls' list of primary goods to include health, by treating health status as a determinant of the range of opportunity open to individuals.

3.1.3 Basic capabilities

Sen (1987) agrees with Rawls' rejection of focusing on utility but criticises his emphasis on primary goods. If it is argued that resources should be devoted to people in poor health, despite there being no utility argument (because they might be contented) and despite there being no primary goods deprivation (because they have the goods that others have), then the basis for such an argument must lie elsewhere. Sen believes that what is at issue is the interpretation of needs in the form of basic capabilities. He suggests that focusing on basic capabilities is a natural extension of Rawls' concern with primary goods.

Sen's work has been very influential in the debate about why health care is considered to be more important than many other commodities. For example, Culyer (1990) has argued that health care, through its impact on health, enables an individual to 'flourish'. So people *need* health care that improves their health. Allocating health care in order to achieve the preferred distribution of health (rather than utility) has two important advantages. First, compared to the measurement of utility, there are a number of established methods for cardinal measurement of health. Second, interpersonal comparisons of health gains can be made from the normative standpoint that a given health improvement is assigned the same value irrespective of the preferences or other characteristics of those involved.

Thus, in the case of distributing health care, what matters is *not* an individual's subjective assessment of their own utility from health care but rather society's assessment of the improved health that health care may produce. Because health is considered to be a basic capability that determines the extent to which a person can flourish, the distribuendum is not utility but basic capabilities (or some health-related sub-set of capabilities).

3.2 *How* is it to be distributed?

Once the distribuendum has been defined, consideration must be given to how it is distributed across people. This section considers alternative conceptions of what the preferred distribution of whatever entities are to be distributed looks like—be it utility, primary goods, or health.

3.2.1 **Sum-ranking**

One way in which we could choose between alternative distributions would be to look at the total amount of well-being generated by each one. The utilitarian philosophy aggregates utility across individuals according to this sum-ranking rule; that is, it looks only at the sum-total of utilities, justified by 'the greatest happiness principle'. As a result, even the tiniest gain in the total sum would be taken to outweigh distributional inequalities of the most blatant kind. For example, would an equal split of 50 to each of two individuals be considered inferior to a situation where one individual had 10 and the other 91, simply because the sum-total of 101 is higher than 100? This particular consequence of the sum-ranking rule is seen (by Rawls, Sen, and others) as violating most reasonable concepts of justice.

However, it is worth remembering that Bentham was in favour of radical redistribution—to argue that each person counts for only one in eighteenth-century Britain was radical indeed. If it is assumed that there is diminishing marginal utility of income, then redistribution from rich to poor will bring about a gain in the sum total of utilities. Note, however, that this concern for distribution is not part of the aggregation rule as such but rather it comes from assumptions that are made about the shape of an individual's utility function.

When the distribuendum is defined in terms of health, it seems that a principle of maximizing aggregate health is not so objectionable—at least not so far as public policy is concerned. The health policy statements of many governments (including those in Norway and the UK) suggest that generating health is one of the most important objectives of the health care system and economic evaluation techniques, such as cost-effectiveness analysis, are designed to provide information so that resources can be allocated to maximize health. The objective of health maximization would mean that an individual's *need* for health care is defined according to their (expected) *capacity to benefit* from that care; that is, the greater their expected benefits, the greater their need.

An allocation of resources 'to each according to their potential for improvement' would mean that a person's pre- and post-intervention *levels* of well-being have no moral relevance in themselves; rather, it is only *changes* in well-being that would matter. This is what advocates of 'maximin' object to.

3.2.2 **Maximin**

Rawls (1971) argues that 'social and economic inequalities must be to the greatest benefit of the least advantaged'. This he refers to as the 'difference principle' although many people now refer to it as 'maximin'. Maximin is a lexicographic principle in that alternative arrangements are compared first from the interests of the least advantaged only. If they are equally as badly off under these arrangements then attention switches to the second least advantaged, and so on.

Since the maximin principle owes much to the work of Rawls, it is concerned with the distribution of primary goods, rather than utility or health. However, as with sum-ranking, it is entirely reasonable to consider the implications of maximin for any given distribuendum. For example, if the concern were with the distribution of health, then resources would be allocated so as to maximize the health of the most severely ill person. The maximin principle would therefore mean that an individual's *need* for health care is defined according to their *severity of illness*. The lexicographic nature of this principle means that resources would be devoted to the most severely ill individual.

Although this decision rule would only apply so long as the expected benefit to the worst-off individual is positive (because 'there can be no duty to do the impossible' (Elster 1992)), it would apply irrespective of the benefits foregone by others, even the next worst-off individual. And so the maximin principle can be criticised for its lack of interest in the magnitude of gains and losses in the chosen distribuendum, and even in the numbers involved.

3.2.3 Egalitarianism

The term *general* egalitarianism is often used when the distribuendum is income whilst *specific* egalitarianism refers to the view that there ought to be an equal distribution of a particular good. However, independently of whether it is general or specific, egalitarianism is referred to as being 'strong' when the preferred solution is the one with the most equal distribution of the distribuendum. Strong egalitarianism can be distinguished from the egalitarianism of maximin that allows for inequalities so long as they benefit the worst off. For example, strong egalitarians would prefer an equal split of 50 units (of utility, primary goods, well-being, and so on) to each of two individuals to a situation where one individual had 90 and the other 51. This is because the latter situation is more unequal (90 and 51) than the former (50 and 50), even though the worst-off individual would benefit from having 51 rather than 50.

Elster (1992) refers to strong egalitarianism as 'strongly envious' but, whilst it may represent an extreme distribution rule, it is not absurd and

does not have to be explained by envy. For example, children often interpret justice as synonymous with absolute equality and many adults may
have a strong aversion to the relative frustration that some people may feel
from having unequal shares.

However, when the distribuendum is no longer income but health,
strong egalitarianism would be absurd in a policy context. It suggests that
a situation in which two individuals are in an equally bad health state is
considered better than the situation in which only one is in that state and
the other is fit and healthy. Hence, at least in the context of health, maximin
emerges as a more sensible rule than strong egalitarianism. In any event, in
the following analysis, the maximin principle and strong egalitarianism
recommend the same distribution of utility (or whatever) so long as the
UPF has a downward slope.

3.3 Choosing a preferred distribution

In what follows, we will consider different distributions of utility between
two individuals, Alan (A) and Bob (B). An identical analysis could be used
for any distribuendum provided that it can be represented by a cardinal
index that allows for unit comparability; that is, the *differences* in each
individual's well-being can be compared with one another.

3.3.1 Choosing a point on the utility possibility frontier

Figure 3.1 shows a UPF that depicts different combinations of maximum
attainable utility for A and B. The UPF is concave to the origin because of
the assumption of diminishing marginal utility (see Chapter 2). This particular UPF is symmetric around the 45° line to reflect the assumption that
A and B have identical preferences.

In such circumstances, sum-ranking, maximin and strong egalitarianism
all recommend the same distribution; that is, an equal one. At point E, the
sum of individual utilities is maximized, the utility of the worst off is maximized, and both individuals have the same utility ($U_A = U_B$ anywhere on
the 45° line but E is the highest point that is attainable on the line).
Therefore, all three rules prefer precisely the same distribution of utility
when there is diminishing marginal utility and when people have identical
preferences.

In order to show how different theories prefer different distributions,
we shall relax the assumption of identical preferences, which is certainly
the more restrictive of the two assumptions. Assume that Alan is able to

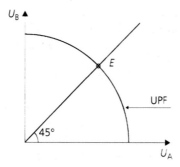

Fig. 3.1 A symmetric utility possibility frontier.

generate more utility from the goods and services he consumes than Bob i.e., he is 'a more effective pleasure machine'. The UPF would then look something like that shown in Fig. 3.2. Utilitarians would prefer the distribution represented by point U where the total sum of utilities is maximized, whilst the Rawlsian-type maximin solution would be at point R where $U_A = U_B$.

Utilitarians would justify U by reference to 'the greatest happiness principle', that is, so long as the loss to the worst off is less than the gain to the better off, the total sum of utility increases. Rawlsians would justify R on the grounds that it is the distribution that maximizes the utility of the worst off. Whether U or R represents the preferred distribution, then, depends on judgements about how utility gains to Alan compare with utility losses to Bob.

One way in which this judgement can be made is to detach people from their own self-interest by concealing their precise position in society. The idea of an *original position* is based upon a view of *justice as impartiality* that argues that an acceptable view for society should reflect agreement between the members of that society. In order to ensure that people's moral decisions are impartial and free from considerations about their own self-interest, Harsanyi (1955) and Rawls (1971) propose a thought experiment where people choose the principles of justice for their society from behind a *veil of ignorance*. This methodology for choosing between different distributions is referred to as *contractarianism* because each individual from behind the veil agrees to sign up to a social contract, and then the veil is lifted.

By assuming that preferences satisfy the axioms of expected utility theory and that the same weight is assigned to all individuals behind the

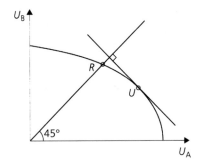

Fig. 3.2 An asymmetric utility possibility frontier.

veil of ignorance, Harsanyi provides justification for the utilitarian solution, U. The Rawlsian veil is a much thicker one in the sense that individuals behind it are deprived of any information relating to the likelihood of them ending up in a particular position. This is because the factors that determine the position people end up in (such as talent and the capacity for effort) vary between people and because even the distribution of those factors is not known behind the veil. According to Rawls, this means that people will fear the consequences of being the worst-off individual and will therefore choose the Rawlsian solution, R.

The veil of ignorance has been the subject of much debate in the literature. Suffice to say here that the operational device of a veil of ignorance does not in itself determine the preferred point on the UPF. It does, however, raise the possibility that other points on the UPF besides U and R might represent the preferred distribution. For example, people may give greater (but not exclusive) weight to the well-being of the worst off. The preferred distribution would then lie somewhere between U and R. According to Elster (1992), it is between these points that we find distributions that appeal to 'the commonsense conception of justice'. The next section considers how the precise point between U and R might be determined.

3.3.2 **The social welfare function**

For many allocation decisions it seems reasonable to assume that people would consider both the size of the gains (however defined) and the likely distribution of those gains. The relative weight that they give to these twin considerations will depend on the extent of their equity–efficiency trade-off; that is, the extent to which they prefer equal shares to a greater overall gain. One way in which to determine this trade-off is to specify a social welfare function (SWF). Most specifications of the SWF assume a constant elasticity of substitution, which means that the curvature or concavity of the curves is constant:

$$W = [\alpha U_a^{-r} + \beta U_b^{-r}]^{-\frac{1}{r}}, \quad U_a, U_b \geq 0, \quad \alpha + \beta = 1, \quad r \geq -1, \quad r \neq 0, \quad (3.1)$$

where W = the level of overall population welfare, that is, the 'social welfare', U_a and U_b = the level of utility (or whatever the distribuendum is) of A and B, α and β = the weight given to one individual relative to the other, as reflected in the *steepness* of the iso-welfare curves, and r = a parameter which measures the degree of aversion to inequality between A and B, as represented by the *convexity* of the iso-welfare curves.

If both individuals are considered to have equal weight, then $\alpha = \beta = 1/2$, thus resulting in contours that are symmetric around the 45° line. This would be the case when neither of them have any distinguishing extraneous characteristics which would justify treating them differently. In deciding whether to treat them differently, Broome (1991) suggests that we look for a class of reasons, referred to as claims, why one person should be given priority over another. He argues that fairness is about mediating the claims of different people and requires that claims should be satisfied in proportion to their strength. (The issue of claims in the context of health care will be returned to in Chapters 5 and 8.)

The parameter r measures the strength of preferences relating to inequality, that is, how close to the equality point R that the preferred location lies. If $r = -1$, social welfare is equal to the sum of individual utility and thus there is *no* aversion to inequality. This utilitarian-type SWF results in iso-welfare curves that are parallel straight lines with a gradient of $-\alpha/\beta$. In eqn 3.1, when the two individuals have equal weight, it follows that social welfare is maximized simply by summing their individual utilities.

If $r > -1$, then there is aversion to inequality, that is, the greater the inequalities between Alan and Bob, the greater is the weight given to the worst-off individual relative to the better-off individual. This results in iso-welfare curves that are *convex* to the origin. In the extreme, the worst-off individual is all that matters and r takes a value of infinity. This will result in a Rawlsian-type SWF with L-shaped (or right-angled) iso-welfare curves. Thus, the higher the parameter value of r, the stronger is the preference for equality, that is, the closer one gets to point R (and, hence, the further away from point U). Figure 3.3 shows these various SWFs (all with $\alpha = \beta = 1/2$).

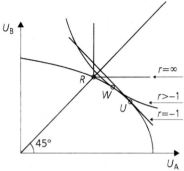

Fig. 3.3 Alternative social welfare optima.

This discussion of distributive justice has located three analytically different points on the UPF, all of which are equally good according to the Pareto criterion. These points are U, the sum-ranking solution suggested by utilitarians; R, the maximin solution associated with Rawls; and W, a trade-off solution following from a SWF which makes trade-offs between the arguments of the former two (corner) solutions. The actual location of this third point critically depends on the degree of aversion to inequality.

3.4 **Alternatives to distributive justice**

3.4.1 **Rights**

Utilitarianism evaluates every action according to the consequent states of affairs. This means that in the context of the debates about the importance of rights, it judges any right according to what happens as a result of the exercising of that right. In this way, it is possible to trade-off different rights against one another in different contexts and, as such, no one right is considered of more intrinsic value than any other. In other words, rights merely serve as rules that should be put in place so as to maximize good consequences. In principle, this makes specifying which rules to enforce a simple task, although, in practice, problems of strategic coordination may arise in devising effective rules. However, this 'utilitarianism of rights' may have some unnerving consequences. For example, it would permit the torture of one person so long as this prevented the torture of someone else (who experienced the same utility loss as a result) and brought about some trivial gain in someone's utility.

Non-consequentialist (or deontological) theories assert that the moral force of rights is not exhausted by their instrumental value. Many such theories judge some rights to have greater moral value than others. For example, possibly the most famous deontological philosopher of them all, Emmanuel Kant (1785), viewed autonomy (the right to rational self-legislation) as perhaps the central moral value. More recently, Nozick (1974) has argued that individuals have certain inviolable rights, such as the right to the fruits of their own labour, which must be respected no matter what their consequences are in terms of the distribution of income. However, this lack of a trade-off between different rights and between rights and other good things has been criticised by many philosophers and economists. As Elster (1992) points out 'In Nozick's theory, distributive issues have *no* independent weight. If liberties and duties are respected, whatever distribution emerges spontaneously will *ipso facto* be just' [italics in original].

Sen and Williams (1982) have suggested a way in which rights could be accounted for whilst still retaining a consequentialist framework. To do this, they allow the evaluation of a state of affairs to differ according to the perspective of the person carrying out the evaluation. So, one torture plus a small gain in utility is better than one torture from a neutral viewpoint but not from the viewpoint of the person being asked to carry out the latter torture. For public policy purposes, most evaluations will take place from a neutral viewpoint, and so a consequentialist framework might be the most appropriate one.

Having said that, there may still be a tension between different principles at the policy level. Take, for example, 'the impossibility of the Paretian liberal' originally discussed by Sen, which shows how considerations of rights might come into conflict with the Pareto principle. In the example, a prude and a lewd are asked for their preferences relating to the censorship policy for Lady Chatterley's Lover. The prude does not wish to read the book but desires even more strongly that the lewd does not read it. The lewd wishes to read the book but would prefer for the prude to read it. The right of self-censorship suggests that it is the lewd who reads the book, but the Pareto principle suggests that it is the prude who reads the book since both individuals would be better off if this were the case.

It could be argued that rights do not conflict with the Pareto principle if individual preferences are based on 'good self-interested reasons' (in this case, over only their own reading decisions) and, whilst it remains a value judgement about what constitutes good self-interested reasons, there is certainly no moral requirement that preferences about other people's activities should be accorded the same moral status as those regarding one's own actions. The paradox and possible ways out of it suggest that, in deciding on the role that preferences should play in determining priorities in health and elsewhere, we need to examine the motivation behind preferences. This is a theme we will return to.

3.4.2 Procedural justice

The discussion in Sections 3.1–3.3 above has considered distributive justice. Consistent with conventional economic thinking, it has focused on outcomes and ignored the means by which a given outcome is achieved. This abstraction can be criticised on the grounds that an individual's welfare may not only depend on the consequences of a policy but on the policy itself. This suggests that, in addition to distributive justice, we need to look at procedural justice, which posits that the fairness of the procedures used in a decision-making process will influence an individual's reaction to the decision. Procedural justice does not deny that the outcome of a decision affects an individual's reaction, but that the process has an effect *independent* of the outcome.

There are two main areas in which a large body of literature on procedural justice exists. The first is law, where 'due process' is of utmost importance in most civil and criminal trials throughout the world. The process—being tried in open, being judged by one's peers, the right to a defence lawyer and so on—takes precedence over any consequences that might result. Now, of course, a fair process might be important precisely because it is considered to produce a fair outcome; that is, trial by jury is the most effective way of making sure that the guilty are convicted and that the innocent are set free. In this way, process is merely instrumental to a fair outcome. But might a fair and transparent process not have intrinsic value? Much of the debate about whether to allow some cases in the UK to be tried by a judge rather than by a jury has focused on the accountability of the legal system and not on its likelihood of making the correct decision.

The second area where procedural justice has made an important contribution is in the literature on participatory democracy. If a process of dialogue whereby all citizens can participate on an equal footing is in place, then the outcome of the democratic process will be deemed to be fair. This can be seen as a kind of rights-based approach in that individuals are held to have inviolable rights to participate in public dialogue. Habermas (1984) has suggested that such dialogue—in which people participate in uncoerced discussion—should be used to choose between alternative theories of distributive justice.

Levanthal (1980) has identified six justice rules that are presumed to govern the evaluation of procedural fairness:

(1) consistency—decisions are deemed to be consistent with one another if the same procedures were applied across different people and over time;

(2) bias suppression—this refers to the absence of vested interests, where individuals who may have personal interests in particular outcomes are excluded from the decision-making process, or at least the potential for bias arising from their involvement is suppressed;

(3) accuracy—the information used in the decision-making process is appropriate and accurate;

(4) correctability—there are mechanisms in place that allow decisions to be challenged or even reversed;

(5) representativeness—this rule provides a platform for individuals to make their opinions known to decision makers;

(6) ethicality—the mechanisms by which decisions are made coincide with the ethical and moral beliefs of those affected by those decisions (for example, the gathering of certain genetic information might be considered to be unacceptable).

Whilst these rules have been most often applied to decision contexts which affect identified individuals, such as in the legal system, they are equally applicable to decisions that affect unidentified people, such as in the allocation of health care resources at the macro level. Although this book deals primarily with issues relating to distributive justice, it will often be important when considering any final distribution to consider the procedures by which that distribution came about.

3.4.3 Medical ethics: different principles at the bedside?

It is important not to lose sight of the context within which all of these debates take place, that is, how to do the most good with limited resources. Such resource-allocation decisions can be made at a number of different levels, from decisions at the macro level to choices between individual patients at the micro level. This raises the question of which level a theory of justice is developed at, and asks us to consider whether different theories might be applicable at different levels.

Deductivism directs attention away from the level of specific judgements, and adopts a 'top-down' approach that emphasizes general rules and principles. Inductivism, on the other hand, adopts a 'bottom-up' perspective that emphasizes the role of specific and contextual judgements in shaping general norms and theory. Coherentism moves in both directions and allows for the refinement of general rules in the light of specific judgements. Rawls adopted this 'third way', and used the term *reflective equilibrium* to refer to the process by which considered judgements are adjusted so that they coincide with the premises of theory. He argued that the difference principle (that is, maximin) was not meant to apply in particular cases, such as when a doctor is choosing between individual patients.

The literature on medical ethics has tended to focus on dilemmas at the bedside, including such issues as when to withdraw treatment, whether to allow abortions, and ethics of assisted suicides and voluntary euthanasia. The two main principles in medical ethics have been *non-maleficence*, that is, the principle of 'do no harm' and *beneficence*, that is, the principle that the potential benefits to a patient must be balanced against the potential risks. More recently, attention has also been focused upon respect for *autonomy*, that is, the principle of respecting the decision-making capacities of patients, and increasingly on *justice*, that is, the principle of distributing benefits, risks, and costs fairly. As a result of such considerations of fairness, there is an increasing recognition in the medical ethics literature of issues focusing on interpersonal comparisons, and on resource allocation at higher decision-making levels.

Before moving on, it is worth noting that medical ethics often focuses on the *virtues* of the agents who make decisions. This contrasts with the theories of justice discussed so far in this chapter, which concentrate on the *obligations* that agents have to behave according to a particular set of principles (such as to maximize utility in the case of utilitarianism). A virtue is a trait of character—a moral virtue being a trait that is morally valued—and this allows us to draw attention to an agent's motivations as well as to their actions. People who are motivated by compassion, for example, would meet our approval, whilst others who act in precisely the same way but from different motives would not. Some medical ethicists have argued that replacing the virtuous judgements of health care professionals with obligation-focused theories will not result in better decision making.

3.5 **Conclusion**

The 'ethics of economics' owes much to the utilitarian philosophy. When economists are accused of being preoccupied with efficiency and maximization issues, they can at least justify this obsession by reference to an important philosophical school of thought. There are two different sets of arguments against this utilitarian conception of justice and fairness. The first argues in favour of alternative points *on* the UPF than the utilitarian sum-ranking point. The suggested alternative points would reflect some notions of equity. These could be based on a Rawlsian argument of maximizing the utility of the worst off, a preference for equal distribution of goods, or preferences for an intermediate point that would balance the twin aims of maximizing the total sum of utilities and of having an equal distribution. Still, while disagreeing with the utilitarian solution, these alternatives have a consequensialistic focus.

The second set of arguments against utilitarianism share a basis in procedural justice. Important here are various notions of citizens' rights. People appear to have a wide range of conceptions on what it involves to consider human beings as being equally entitled to—and worthy of—care. Furthermore, most of us would require that legal justice and democratic principles have been followed. Interestingly, it might well be an implication of a procedural justice argument to opt for a point *inside* the UPF. However, economists normally disapprove of points inside the frontier, because they are Pareto inefficient. We believe that the main reason why economists have problems accepting an interior point is that they do not accept the logic behind the particular procedural justice argument from which the preferred distribution follows. It is indeed a challenge to try and distinguish those inefficient distributions that have an explanation in justice and fairness from those which represent mere waste—and a further challenge to consider whether the price (in terms of foregone benefits) of fair procedures is a price worth paying or not.

One final comment before we move on. Because questions of fairness involve value judgements about the way in which benefits should be distributed, it is sometimes argued that such questions are outside the realm of economics that should instead confine its attention to allegedly value-free efficiency conditions. However, as we hope to have shown in the first part of this book, there are no real qualitative differences between the objectives of efficiency and fairness in terms of their dependence on value judgements. It is our contention, one that provides much of the motivation for the rest of the book, that economics can be made more productive if more attention is paid to the ethical considerations that shape our judgements.

Suggested reading

On the ethical issues at the heart of economics, see Hausman, D. and McPherson, M. (1993) Taking ethics seriously: economics and contemporary moral philosophy. *Journal of Economic Literature*, 31, 671–731.

On the debate about utilitarianism, and for a discussion of the 'impossibility of the Paretian liberal', see Sen, A. and Williams, B. (ed.) (1982) *Utilitarianism and beyond*. Cambridge: Cambridge University Press.

On distributive justice, see Roemer, J. (1996) *Theories of distributive justice*. Harvard University Press, Harvard.

On ethics, see Singer, P. (ed.) (1994) *Ethics*. Oxford: Oxford University Press.

On medical ethics, see Beauchamp, T. L. and Childress, J. F. (2001) *Principles of biomedical ethics*. Oxford: Oxford University Press.

4

Efficiency-motivated responses to market failures

Public intervention in the market for health care is based on two quite separate reasons: 'market failures' and equity. This chapter seeks to analyse the nature of market failures, emphasizing people's selfish motivations for various forms of regulation in the distribution of health care.

This chapter confronts the general model of the perfect market with the more specific characteristics of the market for health care. The context of this inquiry into 'failures' follows the neo-classical economic tradition, where costs reflect all costs to society and benefits are assessed and valued by consumer preferences.

4.1 The perfect market model and the imperfect market for health care

To economists, the perfect market model is a very attractive mechanism for distributing goods and services: consumers get what they want if they pay what things cost. Producers get sufficient revenues to cover the costs of production. Due to the harsh competition between producers, any profits over and above what is needed to keep them in business evaporate in the long run. The marginal social value equals the marginal social costs; that is, the value to society of the last unit of production is the same as the costs to society of producing that unit. Beyond serving as an attractive model, it also serves as a yardstick against which the imperfect real world can be compared with an ideal model world. But what is required for a market to be perfect?

In order to understand why real markets do not always operate so perfectly, Table 4.1 sets out the fairly restrictive assumptions upon which the perfect market model rests.

Even the most 'pro-market' economists admit that not many real world markets satisfy *all* of the above assumptions completely. However, the reason why 'imperfect' markets may still be favoured is that they are

Table 4.1 Some key assumptions behind the perfect market model

Assumption	Implication
(1) Full information	Buyers know how much and when they wish to consume, as well as the quality of the goods
(2) Impersonal transactions	Buyers and sellers act independently and operate at 'arm's length'
(3) Private goods	Only the person consuming the good is affected by it; they pay all the social costs and gain all the social benefits
(4) Selfish motivation	Buyers are 'only in it for getting satisfaction', and sellers are 'only in it for the profit'
(5) Many buyers and sellers	No single buyer or seller can influence the market price, either alone or through coordinated action
(6) Free entry (and exit)	Anyone who would like to sell the products may start to do so, and anyone may leave the market whenever they want
(7) Homogenous products	Buyers cannot distinguish between the products of the different producers

believed to work better than an alternative with public regulation and public ownership. Before considering these issues, though, let us consider the extent to which the market for health care fails to satisfy the assumptions of a perfect market.

1. Individuals do not have *full information* about the timing or costs of illness. This means that planning expenditure on health care, even over a relatively short time period, is almost impossible. This gives rise to insurance markets and an associated set of market failures that are discussed in some detail in Sections 4.2–4.4. Patients also lack information about the quality of health care and about the expected effect of health care on health—this is essentially why they see doctors in the first place. Of course, doctors are not fully informed either, but what is important here is that patients have much less information *relative* to doctors (see Section 4.5).

2. For many health care services, especially in primary care, buyers know who the producer is. The transactions between buyers and sellers are personal and their relationship will be based largely on trust. Thus, the notion

of *impersonal transactions* between atomistic agents is not an appropriate description of the doctor–patient relationship, which is discussed more fully in Section 4.5.

3. Many types of health care are clearly not *private goods*, where benefits are only enjoyed by the person consuming the good. Some preventive health measures such as clean air are quite the opposite; they are *public goods* for which consumption is characterized by *non-excludability* (I can't stop someone else consuming it) and *non-rivalry* (the level of my consumption does not alter someone else's level of consumption). Somewhere in between lies health care for which consumption is characterized by *positive externalities*; that is, one person's health care consumption may positively affect another person's utility. Some of these externalities, and how the market might respond to them, are discussed in Section 4.6.

4. *Selfish motivation* is a controversial, and far from clear-cut, assumption of how consumers and producers behave in the market for health care. Patients may not be so selfish that they disregard any concern with how their condition impacts upon other people. And rarely, if ever, would doctors say that they practise medicine so as to maximize profits—even if they did, a code of professional ethics attempts to restrict them from doing so. In this chapter, we assume that consumers are selfishly motivated whilst Chapter 5 deals with more altruistic reasons for caring for others.

5. As to having large numbers of independent buyers and sellers, there are certainly many buyers of health care (unfortunately, most of us will have to consume some health care at some time), and in most cases we operate sufficiently independently of one another. The numbers of independent sellers will vary. Only in big cities would we find many hospitals but general practitioners and specialists might be found in large numbers and may compete with each other in attracting patients. Overall though, as judged from the assumption of *many sellers and buyers*, the market for health care is imperfect.

Oligopolies (few sellers) and monopolies (one seller) are not unusual features of a market economy because, where there are economies of scale, efficiency will be enhanced by having a smaller number of large producers rather than a larger number of smaller producers. But economic theory considers competition to be good—and monopoly to be bad. This is because monopolies are not 'price-takers' and thus are expected to result in allocative and technical inefficiencies. A profit-maximizing monopolist hospital, for example, will select a higher price and a lower output than a profit-maximizing competitive hospital industry. In addition, monopolistic conditions will result in so-called *X-inefficiencies* (such as managerial slack) due to the lack of incentive to produce at lowest cost, that is, monopolies use more input factors than are necessary for a given output and are thus not on an isoquant (see Chapter 2). The monopolist may try to justify the higher unit costs in terms of increased quality (claiming better health outcomes, for example), but without an adequate measure of patient health outcome (of which more in the next chapter), it may be impossible to distinguish X-inefficiency from genuine quality-enhancing activities.

Whilst cost inefficiencies are expected in monopolistic markets, this conclusion is contingent on the structure of the demand side. If there is full cost reimbursement from insurance, then user-cost is zero and hospitals have an incentive to switch from price to non-price competition in order to attract patients. Higher quality care, more convenient locations, shorter waiting times, and so on, are all cost-raising activities and there is no mechanism for ensuring that any of these dimensions of output are optimal.

6. *Free entry* of providers is not a common feature of the health care market. There are professional regulations that prohibit non-medics from offering their services. In addition, certain types of professional qualifications are required in most countries for practitioners to receive public funding (for example, physiotherapists). And even if they might be prepared to rely on patient payments, many countries regulate the number of various practitioners in any region. However, like in most markets, there is free exit in that doctors may stop practising whenever they want.

There may well be market conditions that prevent competition *in* the market (for example, economies of scale which mean that technical efficiency is achieved through a sole supplier—a natural monopoly) but the idea is to create competition *for* the market. For contracting to work, the bidding environment must be competitive. This does not mean that the market itself has to be competitive. Provided that at least two bidders can offer to provide a specified service and provided that the incumbent hospital (or its management) cannot ignore the threat of entry without risking being replaced by a new producer, then the competitive price and output will result. In other words, the market must be *contestable*. Successful contracting also requires a system whereby bidders' offers can be evaluated—and this requires information. Although price is clearly important in making a decision, it is not the sole criterion by which bids are judged—and this leads us into our last potential source of market failure— different goods.

7. It is quite a common market strategy for providers to attempt to make their products distinguishable from those of their competitors—a practice known as *product differentiation*. The same goes for health care. Although

the chemical substances of drugs from different producers may be *homogenous*, they have brand names, and new and expensive drugs are claimed to be better. Private hospitals and physicians also attempt to make patients believe their services are of a higher quality than those of public providers by wrapping their services in more attractive amenities. Indeed, non-price competition is only possible if patients perceive the services provided by different hospitals or doctors to be different.

In discussing some of the failures in the market for health care in more detail, we will begin by discussing the uncertainties that are inherent in the consumption of health care and highlight some of the problems associated with the health care insurance markets that emerge to deal with these uncertainties.

4.2 Uncertainty and insurance

There are two types of uncertainty in health care that give rise to the development of insurance schemes. First, consumers do not know if they will ever need health care, for example, not knowing if one's house will burn down or one's car will crash. Second, consumers do not know the full financial implications of illness, both in terms of treatment costs and lost earnings. In order to avoid—or at least reduce—the financial uncertainties associated with future illnesses, consumers take out health insurance.

4.2.1 The welfare gain from insurance

Consider an individual without insurance. If the consumer is healthy, they enjoy wealth, W, and if they are ill, they will suffer a 'money equivalent loss', L, thus resulting in wealth, $W - L$. Let the probability of illness be q, and so the probability of not being ill is $1 - q$. Their expected utility, $E(U)$, is their utility from wealth if they are healthy, $U(W)$, multiplied by the probability of them being healthy, plus their utility from the reduced wealth if they are ill, $U(W-L)$, multiplied by the probability of their being ill:

$$E(U) = (1-q)U(W)+qU(W-L). \qquad (4.1)$$

Obviously, the smaller the probability that the illness occurs, and the smaller the expected money loss associated with the illness, the higher is the expected utility.

The welfare gain from insurance can be illustrated by considering the relationship between an individual's wealth and their utility. Figure 4.1 is

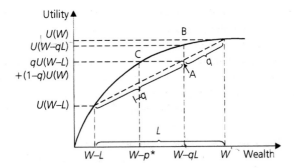

Fig. 4.1 The welfare gains from insurance.

based on the crucial assumption of diminishing marginal utility of wealth (see also Fig. 2.2). W on the horizontal axis represents their wealth when healthy and $U(W)$ on the vertical axis represents their utility from that wealth. $W - L$ and $U(W - L)$ show the corresponding wealth and utility, respectively, when ill. The idea of buying insurance is that the money loss, L, will be compensated for if illness occurs. The cost of this guaranteed compensation is a specified premium, p.

The premium is said to be *actuarially fair* if it represents the insurance company's expected payout; that is, the size of the loss multiplied by the probability of that loss occurring ($p = qL$). When insurance is offered at actuarially fair rates to a large number of people, then the insurance company can expect to pay out the same amount in compensations as they receive in revenues from insurance premiums. Hence, actuarially fair premiums involve no profits and no costs of administering the insurance scheme.

Now, compare wealth and utility with and without insurance. First, the expected wealth is the same. The left-hand side of eqn 4.2 represents wealth *without* insurance and the right-hand side represents wealth *with* insurance (when $p = qL$):

$$q(W - L) + (1 - q)W = W - qL. \tag{4.2}$$

However, as can be seen from Fig. 4.1, the expected utility of wealth is higher with insurance than without it:

$$qU(W - L) + (1 - q)U(W) < U(W - qL). \tag{4.3}$$

Thus, the expected utility represents the probability-weighted average of the utility with and without loss (at point A in Fig. 4.1). On the vertical axis of Fig. 4.1, the utility from the insured situation reflects the point on the utility function corresponding to wealth level $W - qL$. It can be seen that the uninsured situation gives a lower level of utility. Hence, the welfare gain from insurance can be illustrated as *the vertical distance* from A to B between the (expected) utility without insurance and the utility with insurance.

This welfare gain can evaporate with increased insurance premiums. The *horizontal distance* from point A to the intersection of the utility function at point C indicates how much more consumers would be willing to pay for insurance and still remain at the same level of utility as in the uninsured situation. While qL ($=p$) is the actuarially fair premium, p^* (which is larger than p) is the maximum that this consumer would be willing to pay. To the insurance company, $p^* - qL$ represents the maximum 'loading' on insurance, that is, it is the maximum mark-up that an insurance company could charge to cover its administrative costs and to make profit. Thus, if they choose the maximum load factor of $(p^* - qL)/qL$, all the welfare gains from insurance are captured by producers. This may represent an important source of market failure in private insurance markets, and is something we will return to shortly. In the meantime, let us remain under the assumption of actuarially fair insurance contracts.

4.2.2 The probability and the loss

Consider a low probability illness with a large potential loss, q_1L_1, and compare it with a high probability illness with a low loss, q_2L_2. Assume that the *expected loss* of the two illnesses is the same, that is, $q_1L_1 = q_2L_2$. This means that the actuarially fair premium is the same for both illnesses. However, Fig. 4.2 shows that the welfare gain from insurance is highest in the situation with the large potential loss.

The smaller the financial loss, the smaller the welfare gains from insurance. We note that the shorter the vertical distance between the utility curve and the straight line between $U(W)$ and $U(W - L)$, the lower the relative welfare gain from insurance becomes. This is intuitively appealing in that we would be less willing to take out insurance for losses that we could more easily afford. While this explains situations when insurance is not *demanded*, the reduced *supply* of insurance contracts for illnesses with a high probability and a large loss (for example, in the case of some chronic diseases) can be explained by the relatively limited scope for 'loading', and hence the reduced likelihood of covering costs and making profits.

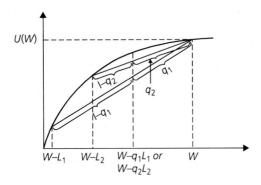

Fig. 4.2 Identical expected losses but different welfare gains from insurance.

So, the market for health care, like other markets, will respond to uncertainty by developing insurance solutions. We have seen that there are efficiency reasons why insurance contracts are not specified for all types of health care. There may be no supply because insurance companies are not able to cover their administrative costs for higher frequency losses and, as a result, contracts cannot be priced low enough for consumers to be willing to take out insurance to cover small losses. In the following, we shall look more closely at market failures in private health insurance.

4.2.3 **Actuarially fair insurance**

Let us begin by considering how a system with unregulated community rating will evaporate. Under this system, *all* consumers/citizens are offered the *same* rate that reflects the expected per-capita loss over the whole community. Using subscript C for community, the premium equals the expected loss, which is the product of the probability of the loss and the size of the loss should it occur, that is, $p_C = q_C L_C$. However, we each have different genetic inheritance and are exposed to different health risks (see Chapter 1). Consequently, each person would have their own expected loss. Imagine that n people can be located on a continuum from the lowest expected loss at one end to the highest expected loss at the other, where $q_C L_C$ represents the community average:

$$q_1 L_1 < q_2 L_2 < \cdots < q_C L_C < \cdots < q_{n-1} L_{n-1} < q_n L_n. \tag{4.4}$$

The feature of this system of community rating is that it involves redistribution *ex ante*, from low-risk to high-risk groups. Again, with a fixed premium, $p_C = q_C L_C$, those with lower than average risk will cross-subsidize those with higher than average risk. The further away from the community average, the larger is the amount of cross-subsidy contributed or received. Clearly, all those with high risks are happy with this system (of course, they may be unhappy with their high risks).

While those with low risks might be happy with this, some might be tempted to opt out and self-insure. To the extent that they are able to signal their lower risks, a second insurance market will develop, where they will be offered cheaper premiums than the current community premium. This *cream skimming* of low-risk groups has some simple arithmetic implications: when low risk individuals leave the group, the average risk (and hence premium) increases for those that remain. Persistent cream skimming will result in each individual paying a tailor-made premium to reflect their own expected loss. Hence, under actuarially fair insurance, there is no redistribution *ex ante*.

The distributional implications of actuarially fair insurance are not market failures as such. High-risk individuals will have to pay high insurance premiums or else pay for health care at the point of delivery. If they cannot afford to do so (which is likely given that high risks are often found in groups with low incomes), then this is an equity, not an efficiency, issue. Rather, market failure in this context relates to the problem that actuarially fair insurance is not possible due to *asymmetric information*. In general terms, this is where an individual or group knows something that other individuals or groups do not. Notice that what is relevant here is the relative amount of information that the individuals have, and not the absolute amount. There are effectively two main types of asymmetric information: *adverse selection* where the asymmetry occurs before the insurance contract is made and *moral hazard* where the asymmetry occurs after the contract is made.

4.3 Adverse selection

Adverse selection arises from population heterogeneity in the risks faced by individuals, combined with asymmetric information about those risks. The heterogeneity is caused by factors that the individual can control (such as certain decisions about their lifestyle) and by factors that they have no control over (such as their genetic inheritance). The problem with actuarially fair insurance is that of signalling and identifying 'true risks'. Sellers of insurance contracts must make sure that the expected loss of a customer is not higher than the premium (plus loading). While they would prefer to charge the highest possible loading, competition among insurance companies will reduce this exploitation of people's dislikes for taking risks (referred to as their *risk aversion*). Buyers would wish to signal that they face a lower risk than they really do, in order to be offered a cheaper premium.

Since buyers may know things that the insurance company does not (or which would be too costly for the insurance company to find out), the problem for sellers is to identify and separate 'false risks' from 'true risks'. One solution is to offer contracts with deductibles (where the insured does not get compensation for losses smaller than some fixed amount) or coinsurance (where the insured only gets a fixed fraction of the losses covered). The market failure of this solution is that it induces self-selection—low-risk buyers will prefer contracts with high deductibles and coinsurance, while high-risk buyers will prefer more complete coverage. Consequently, the less comprehensive contracts are the cheapest because they attract low-risk buyers. In other words, the 'true low risks' have been identified.

However, low-risk buyers might still prefer complete coverage if it were available at actuarially fair rates. But because of false signalling from high-risk buyers, this type of contract would only be offered at a rate that reflects the expected loss of the high-risk group. Hence, low-risk people are faced with the choice between partial insurance at a low rate or full insurance at an excessively high rate. In the absence of actuarially fair and full insurance, low-risk people may choose second-best partial insurance.

Related to adverse selection are inefficiencies from high *transaction costs*. As Culyer (1989) notes, 'Private insurance is bureaucratic and costly, requiring armies of accountants, actuaries, billers, checkers, fraud detectors, lawyers, managers and secretaries'. In fact, administrative costs in the US private health insurance system could account for nearly a quarter of the total costs of health care (Hurley 2000). A single tax-financed system of public insurance is more cost effective when it comes to administrative costs, for four main reasons. First, when 'health taxes' independent of individual risk are included in an existing tax system, there are no additional costs involved with revenue collection. Second, providers of health care face no costs of collecting reimbursements from the insurance companies. Third, there are no costs involved in designing insurance packages for different risk groups. And fourth, there are no advertising costs of the kind found in competitive insurance markets.

The simplest policy solution to adverse selection and high transaction costs, therefore, is compulsory public insurance. It may offer complete coverage without worrying about false signalling and, given economies of scale, is potentially much more efficient when it comes to administration costs. Government insurance certainly involves less consumer choice than private insurance, but it might still be preferred by low-risk individuals who are not offered their preferred choice (that is, full coverage at actuarially fair rates) under private insurance.

4.4 Moral hazard

Moral hazard refers to any tendency for the presence of insurance to increase the probability of loss or its amount. This may result in an individual incurring more expenses with insurance than without it. Now, there is of course a disutility associated with health care, and most of us would prefer to go through our lives without ever having consumed it all. Moreover, there are often substantial non-financial losses associated with poor health—you do not need to pay the costs of a leg fracture, for example, but you would probably still take precautions to avoid the pain and misery of breaking your leg. But still, the existence of insurance may affect an individual's behaviour *at the margin* in that less effort may be taken to avoid the loss. This is referred to as *ex ante* moral hazard.

When the costs of the loss are exaggerated, this is referred to as *ex post* moral hazard. This may be more a problem for health insurance in that it refers to behaviour *after* the sickness has occurred. Patients would prefer a higher level of care (and amenities) when sick than they would if they had to pay for it. Doctors, who tend to have more affinity to the patient in need than to the third party paying the bill, would be prepared to respond by recommending more resources than if the patient had to pay out of their own pocket. This *supplier moral hazard* exists when doctors have a great deal of discretion over the type of care they provide.

The standard—and simplest—model illustrates a situation with constant marginal costs and a downward sloping demand curve that reflects marginal benefits (see Fig. 4.3). With full insurance, a patient would prefer health care up to the point where the demand curve cuts the horizontal axis at a price of zero. Without insurance, the patient would restrict their demand where the curve cuts the marginal cost curve. The shaded triangle between the marginal cost curve and the demand curve illustrates the welfare loss from insurance.

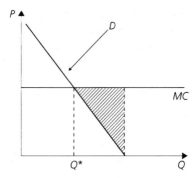

Fig. 4.3 The welfare loss from excess insurance.

Therefore—surprise, surprise—the simple policy solution to this type of *ex post* moral hazard is increased patient payments. The higher the copayment (or coinsurance or cost-sharing), the greater the reduction in the size of the welfare loss triangle. The loss completely disappears, of course, when there is no insurance. The problem with no insurance is that people do not experience the welfare gains from insurance either!

While maintaining the insurance system, there are various policy options to reduce *ex post* moral hazard. Essentially such contracts and treatment guidelines attempt to restrict the choice set of the doctor in such a way that they provide services of the kind that potential patients want *ex ante* rather than what actual patients want *ex post* or what doctors themselves would want.

4.5 Asymmetric information and the agency relationship

Asymmetric information exists when one party possesses more information than the other, and where this information is of a kind that is considered important to the latter. Doctors possess two types of information that are important to patients: diagnostic information ('What is wrong with the patient?') and treatment information ('What can be done for the patient?'). As a consequence, a patient would want their doctor to act as their *perfect agent*. In general terms, an agency relationship exists when one individual or group (the agent) acts on the behalf of another individual or group (the principal). We can consider a doctor as acting as an agent in two distinct ways. First, when they act solely for an individual patient, and second, when they consider other people alongside that patient. For example, they might simultaneously consider their other patients or possibly a third party payer, such as the government or society as a whole.

4.5.1 **The doctor–patient relationship**

The consumption of health care is different from the consumption of most other goods in that the consumer lacks information about the effects that health care will have on their utility. Unlike normal goods that are consumed for their direct utility-yielding properties, health care is consumed for its impact on health. Health care itself is not a 'good' in the conventional sense, but a 'bad' (or a necessary evil) required for improved health. Hence, the demand for health care is a *derived demand* for health. As with most other goods in the utility function, the individual is the best judge of their utility from health. Going back to Fig. 1.1, the consumer is sovereign in judging the utility they get from health directly, as well as indirectly via the impact that health has on wealth and social relations.

However—and this is crucial—the consumer lacks information about the impact of health care on health. Typically, the patient will lack information about which treatments might be available, and the effectiveness of the alternative treatments. In other words, they are relatively ill informed about the production function. On the other hand, the supplier of health care—the doctor—has much greater knowledge concerning the technical relationship between health care and health. Given this information asymmetry, it is not surprising that doctors make decisions on behalf of patients.

Doctors do, however, differ in their views about what it is that patients want from them—some argue that their task is to tell the patient what treatment they should have, others that it is their task to provide the patient with information so that the patient can decide. In theory, this agency relationship is not a problem because the utility function of the agent (the doctor) is identical to that of the principal (the patient)—that of maximizing the utility of each patient. As Williams (1988) points out, if the doctor is the perfect agent, 'The *doctor* is there to give the *patient* all the information the *patient* needs in order that the *patient* can make a decision, and the *doctor* should then implement that decision once the *patient* has made it'.

However, even if patients' and doctors' utility functions were identical (which is unlikely), this still requires that each doctor will have full knowledge of the arguments in each patient's utility function. Now, it seems reasonable to assume that maximizing health will be an objective of most patients and, according to some health economists (see, for example, Culyer 1989; Williams 1988), it is assumed to be the *only* relevant argument in patients' utility functions. However, other arguments such as the amount of information requested or the desired degree of involvement in the decision-making process are likely to be important and will naturally differ across patients. Thus, it is unlikely that any doctor could act as a perfect agent for his patient.

In reality, the agency relationship that has evolved in health care is one in which the supplier can greatly influence the consumer's utility function. Because doctors hold a position such that they can have some influence over both the costs and benefits of health care, there is the potential for exploitation. Williams (1988) claims that the more recognizable form of his characterization of the agency relationship is one in which the words 'doctor' and 'patient' are reversed: 'The *patient* is there to give the *doctor* all the information the *doctor* needs in order that the *doctor* can make a decision, and the *patient* should then implement that decision once the *doctor* has made it.'

It seems that the only effective constraints on doctors' behaviour are medical ethics (see Chapter 3), which provide some reassurances that the doctor will attempt to do their best for the individual patient, and clinical guidelines, which aim to reduce the wide differences in medical practice (even if these guidelines are themselves formulated largely from existing practice patterns). However, because the choice of treatment recommended by the 'seller' may have many important consequences for the 'buyer', the latter is better described as a vulnerable patient rather than as an empowered consumer. So, the market for health care clearly violates the assumption of impersonal market transactions—buyers and sellers are almost hugging one another rather than operating at arm's length. And because the doctor–patient relationship is so heavily based on trust, the doctor could exploit the patient in a variety of ways—possibly even inducing demand that might not otherwise exist.

4.5.2 Supplier-induced demand

Supplier-induced demand (SID) refers to the extent to which a doctor provides or recommends the provision of medical services that differs from what the patient would have chosen if they had the same information and knowledge available as the doctor. According to the authors of a US-focused health economics textbook, 'No single issue in the relatively brief history of health economics has generated more interest and controversy than supplier induced demand' (Folland *et al.* 1997). Whilst SID has not generated the same level of attention from European health economists, it still has important implications for less market-oriented health care systems.

Supplier-induced demand arises from the simple fact that many remuneration systems of doctors are designed so that the more services they provide to each patient, the more income they generate. Indeed, SID is inextricably linked with other theories such as the 'target income hypothesis', which reduces the motivation for imperfect agency behaviour down to income. However, this is a rather narrow view, since the agent seeks to maximize *utility*, of which income will be only one part. As a result, other arguments in the agent's utility function can be the 'trigger' for imperfect agency.

The positive debate on SID has dealt with the issue of whether doctors have the power to shift the demand curve further out in the price–quantity space, and how the eventual extent of this inducement could be tested empirically: 'Can we ever really know its extent?' (for a funny parable on this, see Fuchs 1986). This question has been answered using *macro* and *micro* tests. The main macro test to date has been to look at the effect of a change in the population–physician ratio on doctors' fees and the use of services. Typically this is undertaken by using cross-sectional data. As different areas may produce different utilization rates or fee levels for reasons other than physician supply, data on other factors are also used to control for potential confounding factors.

The hypothesis is that doctors, behaving entirely rationally, respond to an increase in the supply of doctors by generating greater demand for their services to maintain their target level of income. There is plenty of evidence to suggest that there is a positive relationship between supply of doctors and the use of medical services. The evidence on the relationship between the supply of doctors and fees is less conclusive. For example, an increase in the utilization of medical services following an increase in supply is consistent with standard economic theory if price falls, and a positive relationship between the supply of medical services and price points to a shift in demand.

Micro tests of SID concentrate on doctors' responses to financial incentives by looking at how doctors respond to fee controls or to a change in their method of remuneration. The hypothesis being tested is that both fee controls and a change in methods of remuneration will lead to a change in the quantity of services being provided as doctors attempt to maximize their income or utility or maintain their target income. Such 'natural experiments' do not have many of the drawbacks of the macro tests, for example, typically there are better quality data and fewer confounding factors. These tests provide compelling evidence of physicians changing their level or type of services provided in line with predictions from the target income hypothesis.

As an excellent example, Krasnik *et al.* (1990) looked at the provision of general practitioner (GP) services in Denmark. In Copenhagen, GPs were paid a fixed rate (that is, on a *capitation* basis) whilst their counterparts elsewhere were paid on a mixed capitation/fee-for-service basis. The income of GPs in Copenhagen fell, and so they demanded a change in remuneration. Services in and out of Copenhagen were studied before the change and twice after. Three hypotheses were tested. First, GPs in the city would increase their overall activity after the change. Second, referrals to specialists and hospitals would decrease after the change. And third, in the short term, doctors would be more likely to overshoot their target income but thereafter their overall activity would fall as they could attain their target incomes.

The results suggested that activity did increase after the change and that referrals did decrease as GPs took the opportunity to undertake many now more lucrative services for themselves. The level of activity fell between the second and third rounds after the initial increase between the first and second rounds. All of this is suggestive of SID.

The normative debate about SID has dealt with the extent to which we can accuse doctors of doing such bad things—since almost by implication SID is a bad thing—for patients. Whether or not SID really is a bad thing has a simple analytical answer, namely, if the demand has been shifted to the right of the point where the initial (and assumed autonomous) demand curve hits the horizontal quantity line (see Fig. 4.3). If it has not, this partial model suggests that a revenue-maximizing doctor has not done anything morally wrong to the patient. Whether or not SID is morally wrong for society depends on whether or not demand has been pushed to the right of the point at which *society's* valuation of marginal benefits is lower than social costs (at Q^*), something which is more likely to happen.

We suggest here that it is reasonable to conclude that some demand inducement exists—we might not be able to see it but we can certainly smell it and taste it. The shift in the demand curve is symptomatic of an imperfect agency relationship arising out of *asymmetric information*, which gives the doctor some discretion in their decisions, and *personal transactions*, which means that the doctor can persuade the patient to trust those decisions. This is not withstanding the fact that the code of medical ethics outlined in Section 3.4.3—nonmaleficence, beneficence, autonomy, and justice—will act as a powerful constraint on the profit-maximizing behaviour of doctors and other health professionals. And, as also discussed in Section 3.4.3, suppliers may be motivated by a moral duty towards their patients.

Anyhow, the fact that doctors, like everyone else, respond to pecuniary and non-pecuniary incentives is no bad thing. It means that with the right incentives, we can get doctors to behave how we would like them to behave. Thus, if we first establish how we want doctors to behave, then assess the nature of the doctor's utility function and investigate their responses to changes in incentive structures, we can finally design structures to induce doctors to behave efficiently. And so the existence of SID—the result of selfish motivation—might not be so bad after all.

4.5.3 The agency relationship and social welfare

Discussions of the individual doctor–patient relationship appear to suggest that a perfect agent is a doctor who provides the patient with the combination of services that is most preferred by the patient themselves. However, what the patient wants might differ from what society wants the patient to have. For example, in the consultation room, a patient might want all the beneficial health care there is, irrespective of its cost. They might also want the most expensive and luxurious amenities. However, as a payer for health care *ex ante*, they might be willing to contribute towards only that part of health care that contributes directly to health rather than to utility more generally. This kind of paternalistic altruism can be explained by the various types of externalities in health (discussed in Section 4.6 and Chapter 5).

This raises general questions about what the maximand of health care is and about what the objectives of the health sector are. It also raises more specific questions about who the doctor is ultimately the agent for—the patient, a group of patients, those funding health care, or society as a whole? Doctors, like the rest of us, cannot please all of the people all of the time, and so the answers to these questions will determine what the perfect agent looks like.

Consider the following framework which, following the medical code of ethics that 'the health of my patient shall be my first consideration', is based on the assumption that doctors should act in the best interest of the patients *ex post*. This is against a background that those who contribute towards health care may have two sets of preferences—one about the services they would like for themselves should they become ill and one about those services which they are prepared to contribute towards for others. The idea comes from Evans (1984) who suggested that people might prefer complete discretion over their own care yet feel paternalistic about the care of others.

Within this framework, it can be shown that the size of the health care budget depends on the choices made by doctors regarding the mix they offer between health-enhancing services and those services which have no impact on health but which patients may still want for other utility-enhancing reasons. If doctors provide a mix that reflects the preferences of patients *ex post*, those providing funding will react by reducing their contributions to health care since they do not like to see health care being 'wasted' on services that do not improve health. However, the very same providers of funding would still wish to see such services being available to themselves should they end up as patients.

Given such *split preferences*, doctors will act in accordance with the *ex-ante* preferences of their patients if they provide *less* non-health-enhancing services than those very same patients would prefer. By restricting 'waste', the total health care budget is increased, thereby enabling doctors to treat more patients (for an elaboration of this model, see Clark and Olsen 1994). This model is based on an assumption that our willingness to cross-subsidize health care depends on the effectiveness of that care in improving health. This assumption will be set in a wider context below, and is discussed more fully in Chapter 5.

4.6 **Externalities—selfishly motivated**

Assuming that health care represents a private good would imply that nobody beyond the consumer/patient themselves benefits from the use of health care. However, an inquiry into the various types of interpersonal relationships in health suggest that there are four different ways in which the improved health that a person obtains from their health care use may affect another person's utility. Economists refer to the impact of one person's behaviour on another person's utility as an *externality*. Externalities in the use of health care are illustrated in Fig. 4.4, which represents an extension of Fig. 1.1.

Figure 4.4 illustrates the case for two individuals, A and B. The focus is on how B's improved health may affect A. As an extension of Fig. 1.1,

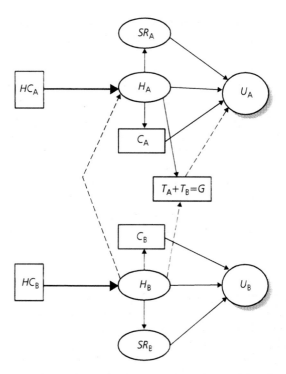

Fig. 4.4 The interpersonal relationships in health. *HC*, health care; *H*, health; *C*, consumption; *T*, tax; *G*, government spending (public goods); *SR*, social relations; *U*, utility.

the wealth (W) is sub-divided into own consumption (C) and tax contributions (T) that go to finance government spending (G), that is, public goods such as schools, parks, and defence. So, why would A care about B's use of health care (and vice versa, which for expositional reasons are not drawn in this figure)? There are two *selfish* reasons that will be dealt with here, and two *altruistic* reasons that will be discussed in Chapter 5.

4.6.1 Contagion

Contagion is illustrated in Fig. 4.4 by the dotted arrow from H_B to H_A. This refers to health care consumed by B which may have a positive impact on A's health, such as vaccination and the cure of infectious diseases. In an unregulated market, B will consume this type of health care (like any other) up to the level where their private benefits equal costs. However, in a societal perspective, this is not sufficient due to the existence of *positive externalities*, which imply that A (along with all other affected fellow members of society) will experience benefits beyond B's individual benefits. These benefits—as valued by the rest of society—should be added to the individual benefits in order to derive *aggregate social benefits*.

So, how can such market failures be corrected for—how can the externalities be internalized? The simple answer is for the rest of society to cross-subsidize B's costs of these services to the extent that they will face private costs which are so low that they will choose to consume the socially optimal quantity. To illustrate this, let us assume that an individual's private benefit (PB) is given by their maximum willingness to pay for health care. The external benefits (EB) are those that are valued (again through a willingness to pay) by other people besides the consumer. Therefore, the summation of PB and EB represents social benefits (SB). Let us also assume that all relevant social costs (SC) are included. The optimal amount consumed is where $SB = SC$ (see also Fig. 2.10):

$$PB + EB = SB = SC. \tag{4.5}$$

The optimal level of cross-subsidization implies that EB is subtracted from SC. In Fig. 4.5, PB illustrates the private demand curve, and SB represents society's demand curve. Thus, the vertical distance between the two curves reflects EB. For simplicity, we have assumed constant marginal SC. The intersection between PB and SC gives the private quantity, Q_P, which is where the individual would choose to consume in the absence of any influence from others. The intersection between SB and SC gives the socially optimal quantity, Q_S. The individual can be induced to move there if we subsidize health care by the vertical distance between SB and PB at this quantity.

Interestingly, this optimal level of cross-subsidy (that is, the vertical distance between the two benefit curves at the point where $SB = SC$) does not imply that consumers would face a zero price. Analytically, this represents a special case. Figure 4.5 illustrates an optimal solution where the consumer has to pay a positive amount. It is, however, quite possible to imagine situations where the external benefits to the rest of society might be so large that the locus of the intersection between SB and SC might even imply that individual consumers should face a negative private price; that is, they should be paid to consume health care.

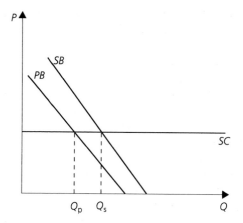

Fig. 4.5 Positive externalities from health care.

Any cross-subsidy could be through voluntary donations, tax financing, or information campaigns or health laws. The growth of public health care is very much a history of fighting contagious diseases, and immunization and vaccination have at various times been provided free of charge.

4.6.2 **Productivity**

An important consequence of improved health is that it affects productive capacity. Not surprisingly, economists have recognized for a long time the importance of healthy labour for economic growth. For example, the early economic evaluation techniques considered the increased value of production from improved health as the way to measure outcomes from treatments—the focus was on repairing an input factor, the human capital. This increased productivity would increase income that in turn increases consumption. In an influential health economic model, these impacts are termed the 'investment benefits' from health, as opposed to the 'consumption benefits' which follow from the enjoyment of being in better health (Grossman 1972).

If increased production ends up as own consumption only, and if we are indifferent to a fellow citizen's consumption level, then there are no externalities from the wealth generated. However, in most economies, some of the increase in an individual's wealth ends up contributing towards society, for example, people pay income tax that goes towards the financing of public goods and services. The self-interested reasons why we are concerned with our fellow citizens' increased economic contributions to society are, first, that public goods and services are positive arguments in our utility function, and second, if a sufficient level of such goods was already produced, then a greater contribution from others means that we will have to pay less ourselves.

Therefore, if the only reason that we cared about the health of others was because of their economic contribution to society beyond their own consumption (the link in Fig. 4.4 between $H_B \rightarrow T_B \rightarrow G \rightarrow U_A$, we would be willing to subsidize their health care so that they could return to the workforce. We would do so as long as the expected future economic contributions exceed the costs of treatment, that is, as long as people 'pay their way' in terms of their use of collective resources ($T_B - HC_B > 0$).

The implication of this type of selfish concern for others is of course that we would provide a higher subsidy to those groups in society who will make the highest economic contributions from being treated. One way that this has been put into practice in some countries is to have sickness benefit funds that pay the costs of treating people who would return to work as a consequence of cure. While this may be a quite rational selfish argument, it might well be that there is a conflict here with one of the key equity objectives of many health systems, namely, 'equal access for equal need', independent of economic position. There will be more on this in the next chapter.

4.7 **Conclusion**

No market works perfectly. But some work less perfectly than others—and the market for health care appears to be one of them. There are a number of reasons for market failure in health care and this chapter has highlighted the most pervasive. In essence, the market fails primarily because of a range of informational asymmetries. Insurers have less information than patients about the risks they face, and patients have less information than doctors about the relative effectiveness of alternative treatments.

There are a number of ways in which the market mechanism can be improved to mitigate the adverse consequences of various kinds of asymmetric information, but every country in the world recognizes that there is the need for considerable government involvement and regulation in the market for health care. It is important to reiterate that this involvement and regulation could be motivated out of a concern for efficiency alone—we might not care one jot about equity and still have government involvement in health care. The discussion of externalities in this chapter has highlighted two of the most important efficiency-motivated responses to market failure. When we add equity and distributional considerations to the picture—which we are about to do in the next chapter— the case for replacing the market mechanism in many parts of health care becomes overwhelming.

Suggested reading

For a standard reference in health economics, see Arrow, K. (1963) Uncertainty and the welfare economics of medical care. *American Economic Review*, 53, 941–73, which has been reproduced, and commented upon, in a special issue of the *Journal of Health Politics, Policy and Law* (October 2001).

We strongly recommend Chapters 2–4 in Evans, R. (1984) *Strained mercy: The economics of Canadian health care.* Toronto Butterworths (available on the web at http://www.chspr.ubc.ca//misc/Strained_Mercy/).

Rice, T. (1998) *The economics of health reconsidered.* Chicago: Health Administration Press.

5

Equity-motivated responses to market failures

There are many reasons why we care for other people's health to the extent that we are willing to subsidize their use of health care. This chapter begins with an inquiry into altruism, before discussing various aspects of equity. Altruism is discussed through the eyes of 'the individual as a consumer', while equity is seen through the eyes of 'the individual as a citizen'.

A market failure in the current context means that people have preferences for a more equal distribution of—and access to—health care than would be created by an unregulated market. We suggest that an egalitarian distributive principle of 'equal access for equal need' may reflect the preferences of the majority of individuals who go to make up society. We consider equity-motivated responses to arise out of a positive concern for the health or well-being of others (rather than, for example, as replacing the market mechanism through a consumer-unfriendly ideology of 'socialized medicine').

So why does (equity-motivated) redistribution take place? The various explanations reflect different political ideologies. To libertarians, all redistribution (other than that based on individual voluntary donations) is *coerced*. They perceive the rich as being forced through the political process and the ballot box to redistribute some of their income to the poor who hold the political power due to majority rule. A Marxist explanation of redistribution would be to consider it as an insurance for the ruling capitalists, who will reduce the probability of revolution by bribing the working class with such things as a minimum income, pensions, and access to education and health care. These rather cynical explanations leave little room for people to genuinely care for one another—either the poor are seen as 'ripping off' the rich or the rich are seen as offering some minimum compensation in return for exploiting the poor.

The third explanation that we shall go into more closely is based on the view that people care about their fellow citizens. The idea of *voluntary* redistribution reflects this altruism and can be analysed within the framework of interdependent utility functions. Set within a two-person world with a rich (R) and a poor (P) person, redistribution involves R giving away some of their income, Y, to P ($-\Delta Y_R = \Delta Y_P$). Voluntary redistribution will continue until R's gain in marginal utility from P's increased income is equal to R's marginal utility loss from his own reduced income.

However, voluntary redistribution may lead to a lower degree of redistribution than that which would be considered optimal by rich people. One reason for this is that 'free-riding' may occur when we extend the model from a two-person to an n-person world. Here, a rich person could watch other rich people contribute towards the poor but, because the marginal benefit to the poor from his own contribution would be small, he might not do likewise himself. In other words, he could 'free-ride' on the backs of the contribution of others. So, it may be rational for rich people to vote for compulsory redistributive taxation so that other rich people do not free-ride. This offers an explanation of why many rich citizens vote for political parties whose tax policies will reduce their own private consumption—an explanation that makes sense only when distinguishing between the individual as a citizen and as consumer. Barr (1993) refers to such behaviour as 'voluntary compulsion'.

Still, this degree of voluntary redistribution (even when decided collectively among the rich to be made compulsory) will only be optimal so far as rich people are concerned. If the rest of the people in society (that is, the poor) are of the opinion that it is fair for the rich to give away more, it follows that voluntary redistribution will produce less equality than that which would result from democratic majority rule.

5.1 Reasons for caring—defining altruism

Altruism is the opposite of selfishness. According to *The Concise Oxford Dictionary* (6th edn) it means 'regards for others as a principle of action'. However, actions that are basically to the benefit of others might also have a 'selfish side-effect'. Equally, actions that are basically selfishly motivated might result in benefits to others. Sen (1987) claims that a mixture of selfish and selfless motivations can explain much of our behaviour in a wider range of social situations. Why, then, do we care about other people and how do we identify actions that have purely selfless motivations?

A first set of explanations for altruism is that the donor gets personal utility from showing sympathy or undertaking actions that they consider to be social duties. In other words, donors 'purchase moral satisfaction' or get 'warm glow' feelings from doing good things. So, in order to obtain the feeling of being a decent citizen, the donor is motivated to act in ways that benefit others. Some economists and philosophers would argue that all altruistic acts must, by definition, bring personal utility—or why else do them?

Adam Smith has been widely quoted as championing self-interest but this is a mistaken view. Despite recognizing that 'self-love' enabled mutually advantageous trade to take place, he did not assign a generally superior role to the pursuit of self-interest. However, much of Smith's writings on the role of ethical considerations in human behaviour have become neglected as these considerations have become unfashionable in economics. This is in spite of the evidence that the success of some free-market economies (such as Japan—well, at least until recently) has been partly based on departures from self-interested behaviour in the direction of duty and loyalty. In any event, defining all actions as being motivated out of self-interest quickly reduces to a tautology that leaves no room for the possibility of genuinely altruistic acts.

Certainly some types of actions that might appear to be altruistic are not so. One type can be explained by *reciprocity*, that is, we do good things for others because we hope and expect that they would do the same in return. This is the mentality of 'I'll scratch your back, if you scratch mine'. Or 'I'll get this round of drinks (... if you get the next round)'. In the former case, I depend on someone else to do something I appreciate (scratch my back), and the price I pay is to do the same thing for that person. In the latter case, it is social convention in some societies to buy drinks in rounds, which serves to reduce the total transaction costs of a night out on the beers (and which may also serve to enhance a sense of group belonging).

While these examples deal with one-to-one reciprocity, the idea of reciprocity can be extended to society, that is, 'I'll do good things for others, because I might rely on my fellow citizens doing good things for me'. In this way, such reciprocity might be seen as investment and insurance for the purposes of creating a supportive social climate that is to the benefit of all. And in this sense, reciprocity is strategic and motivated from concerns other than the direct personal utility from giving *per se*.

Another type of action that might appear to be altruistic is what we refer to as '*conspicuous altruism*'. This is inspired by the concept of 'conspicuous consumption', a term introduced by the (Norwegian-)American economist Thomas Veblen, which refers to how the upper social classes use some types of consumption as means for showing off their excess wealth. The foremost aim of this type of consumption is to signal a successful social position. Analogous to the above concept of 'purchasing moral satisfaction', people can purchase social position through conspicuous consumption. Conspicuous altruism might acquire even greater social status in that donors are seen as doing something good for others rather than as spending excess wealth on frivolous private consumption. The rationale behind making donations conspicuous, then, is that the donors know that they can be identified by the society who will bestow social approval on them.

Some types of actions that benefit others might be to the direct benefit of oneself. Other actions, whose *outcomes* are clearly to the benefit of others, might be influenced by selfishness in the *process* of giving. When we say that we care for the health or well-being of known individuals who are part of our social relations, for example, this might be explained by the fact that we are directly affected by their suffering. Being affected could involve constraints on our own life (for example, caring for a sick child) or could simply result in us being emotionally stressed. We resist using the term altruism when there is such direct benefit.

Is there anything left that we can legitimately call *genuine* altruism? To qualify as genuine altruism an action must not contain any degree of reciprocity, must not involve any element of gaining social approval, and the donor cannot have any personal or social relations with the beneficiaries. Genuine altruism exists when we simply care that other people's well-being has fallen below a level that we consider to be acceptable. Rich and fit people may be observed to care for poor and sick people (particularly when the suffering of the latter is the result of factors outside of their control). Looking back at Fig. 4.4, we can add two altruistic arrows, indicating that individual A may care for the health of individual B ($H_B \rightarrow U_A$) or for B's utility or well-being ($U_B \rightarrow U_A$). The former suggests that subsidies should be in the form of health care while the latter suggests cash transfers.

5.2 Transfers in cash or in kind

There is a spectrum from general altruism to paternalistic altruism defined according to the extent to which the donor respects the preferences of the recipient. At one extreme lies general altruism, which, consistent with the new welfare economics, regards each individual as the best judge of their own welfare. In such cases, the donor is happy for the recipient to do whatever they like with the redistributed income. A transfer in cash will then allow the recipient to maximize their utility. At the other extreme lies paternalistic, or goods-focused, altruism. This involves limiting or changing the choice set of the recipient, usually in line with the preference of the donor.

Consider the following example of a donor's choice of a present, the monetary value of which is constrained by the cost of a compact disc (CD). If a general altruist, the donor would hand over the cash, which the recipient could then spend on anything. A goods-focused altruist, on the other hand, might buy the recipient a particular CD that he ('the pater') thinks the recipient *ought to* listen to. Of course, there are weaker forms of paternalistic altruism. For example, he might buy a gift voucher for the type of music he feels the recipient should listen to (for example, in a classical CD shop). Or alternatively, and closer to the general altruist, the donor might simply feel that the recipient should consume music (of whatever style) and hence might buy a gift voucher from a general CD shop.

It is worth noting here that limiting the choice set of the recipient does not necessarily have to be line with the preferences of the donor. It might well be in accordance with the recipient's best interests as judged by some third party. For instance, we might know that pension savings, social insurance, education, nutrition, housing, and access to health care are all goods that we would like to have available to us. In this sense, such transfers are in accordance with the long-term interests of the recipient. However, it is paternalistic insofar as it involves limiting the *immediate* choice set of the consumer.

In the context of the utility function set out in Fig. 4.4 (which contains own consumption, C_A, own health, H_A, public goods, G, own social relations, SR_A, and others' health, H_B, or utility, U_B), these interpersonal relationships can be expressed in the equations below, where eqn 5.1 illustrates general altruism and eqn 5.2 shows goods-focused (in this case health-focused) altruism:

$$U_A = u(C_A, H_A, G, SR_A, U_B) \tag{5.1}$$

$$U_A = u(C_A, H_A, G, SR_A, H_B). \tag{5.2}$$

A's paternalism towards the health of B could be explained by A's preference that B should live a healthy lifestyle, a kind of 'healthism'. Or it might be that A views B's health as instrumental to his ability to 'flourish' as a human being, so ultimately A is concerned with B's well-being, but believes health is central to that. In either case, A has a stronger preference for health relative to other goods than he thinks B has.

A standard model in economics textbooks is to explain why—in terms of the recipient's utility—transfers in cash are always better than transfers in kind. This should be intuitively obvious: if the money value of an in-kind transfer is handed over as a cash transfer, the recipient can acquire the same in-kind bundle if that is what they want. However, if they choose to spend some—or all—of the money on other goods, then this reveals that they get higher utility from an alternative consumption bundle. Thus, in those cases where the recipient would not choose to spend all of their cash transfer on the good that would otherwise be transferred in kind, a smaller transfer in cash than in kind is required to bring about a given increase in utility.

This 'proof' in favour of cash transfers is based upon an implicit assumption that the donor is a general altruist, that is, the size of his donation is independent of what the recipient spends the transfer on. However, one of the main reasons for in-kind transfers is that the donor (or some third party acting on their behalf) believes that some goods are more important to the recipient's well-being than other goods—and that, when left to their devices, the recipient will go for other goods (which are 'less good' in the eyes of the donor). If the donor's contribution was lower if the transfer was in cash rather than in kind (because they are paternalistic), then the recipient might in fact gain greater utility from a larger transfer in kind than from a smaller one in cash.

Textbooks in economics often refer to the type of goods that are being transferred in kind as 'merit goods'; that is, 'commodities in respect of which the state overrides consumer sovereignty' (Barr 1993). This concept is often extended to distinguish between 'merit goods' and 'merit bads', where the consumption of the former is believed to be good for people and should therefore be subsidized, while the latter is believed to be bad for people and should therefore be restricted or taxed.

The problem with the concept of merit goods (and bads) is that the justification for overriding consumer preferences is unclear. As suggested above, it would seem to be indicative of the morality of the donors or a reflection of a genuine concern for the long-term interest of the recipient, and these are sometimes very difficult to disentangle. There are many economists, philosophers, and lay persons, who possess the rhetoric skills of wrapping their own moral beliefs and prejudices into being consistent with the best interests of other people. In any event, the rationale behind transfers in kind is to limit the choice set of recipients, so as to encourage the consumption of goods or discourage the consumption of bads. The provision of specific health services, rather than providing people with health 'vouchers' which they might then trade on the open or black markets, certainly limits their choices.

Once the preferences of paternalistic donors are included in the calculation of social welfare, along with the preferences of recipients, there is a tension between preserving a central tenet of welfare economics that each individual is the best judge of their own welfare and adopting a position which allows the preferences of the donors—about the recipients' well-being—to dominate. Much of the debate between 'welfarist' and 'non-welfarist' economists revolves around this tension (we have chosen not to use Culyer's (1989) label 'extra-welfarist' as this could imply a particular position which goes beyond welfarism).

Within the bundle of 'merit goods', some will undoubtedly be considered to be more meritorious than others. While health care in general is referred to as a 'merit good', some types of health care are clearly more important in the eyes of the subsidizer. In health policy debates, these are referred to as 'core services'. It is argued that such 'core services' should be subsidized more fully than other types of health care and this is an issue we will return to. For now, the conclusion is that the observed differences in society's willingness to subsidize various types of health care might be explained by different degrees of paternalistic altruism.

5.3 Concerns for more than one individual

So far in this chapter, we have considered caring and sharing in the context of an individual utility function. We have essentially been in a two-person economy with rich and poor. Let us now consider a third person, S, who is also poor. Equation 5.2 can then be changed to:

$$U_R = u(C_R, H_R, G, SR_R, H_P, H_S).\qquad(5.3)$$

A question that arises now is who does R have the greatest altruistic concerns for, P or S? If P and S are equal in all relevant aspects, it is difficult to imagine that R should feel more altruism for one over the other. Hence, R would most likely divide his health care subsidies equally between them: 'equals are to be treated equally'. Still, if all three of them suffered from the same health problem, R might wish to allocate more to their own health care than to the health care of P or S. If they did, R would reveal themselves to be an 'egalitarian free-rider', that is, subscribing to equal access among everybody else but superior access for themselves. (How many of us, we wonder, might not hold such preferences?)

While it is fruitful to discuss altruism towards other citizens within the framework of an individual utility function, this framework makes less sense for discussing preferences over equity principles that include the whole of society. We will therefore move away from the preferences of the individual as a consumer and towards their preferences as a citizen. This distinction owes much to Rousseau (1762), who claims that an individual has two roles in society; one as a private individual and one as a citizen. As a private individual, they are motivated by personal utility, and as a citizen, they are motivated by the utility of the collective. Harsanyi (1955) has suggested that an individual has two sets of preferences—one based on what they personally prefer and one relating to social considerations—which may come into conflict with one another. And Etzioni (1986) has suggested that moral or ethical decisions might require a different utility function because what gives an individual pleasure and what they consider to be 'right' might be mutually exclusive in some circumstances.

The distinction between our roles and motivations as consumers and as citizens represents the second major distinction between welfarism and non-welfarism (that is, in addition to whether or not individuals are seen as the best judges of their well-being). From personal preferences we move to the level where citizens express preferences for distributive principles for health care. This non-welfarist approach, like the welfarist one, respects people's preferences. However, whilst welfarism considers a consumer's preferences to be largely isolated from a social context, the non-welfarism we have in mind here considers a citizen's preferences firmly in the context of social relations. To us, there seems every reason to suppose that the same individual will have different arguments, or at least give different weight to the same arguments, in their utility functions as a consumer and as a citizen.

5.4 **Concerns for the community**

A range of contemporary theories, collectively referred to as communitarianism, focus attention squarely on the 'individual as citizen' since they recognize that individuals are social animals with high social needs rather than free-floating atoms in a social vacuum. It is little wonder, then, that communitarianism developed as a response to liberal philosophies (such as utilitarianism) that, in various ways and to various degrees, place the individual centre-stage in any moral discourse. Communitarians argue that shared obligations come from communal ideals and responsibilities rather than from freely made contracts between individuals.

Communitarians clearly set themselves against rights-based approaches. The question to a communitarian, then, is not 'Does this decision or policy violate autonomy?' but rather 'Is it conducive to a good society?'. In this sense, it appears similar to utilitarianism that is concerned with the total utility generated by an action or decision rule. However, communitarians reject the concept of utility on the grounds that it is removed from decision making which affects communities—and, besides, it is too individualistic to sum individual costs and benefits.

Communitarianism can take many forms and has sometimes been categorized as militant and moderate, depending on how hostile the theory is to individual rights. We will not distinguish between the two here; rather, we will highlight those common themes that are relevant to our discussion about why we care about others. Communitarian theories emphasize the importance of exchange between individuals and the communities to which they belong. Individuals have duties to their communities (such as to obey the law) and communities have duties to the individuals within them (such as to preserve the family unit).

With duties come claims—if someone is able to make a legitimate claim to health care (on the grounds of clinical need, say), then someone else has a duty to provide it (for a discussion of claims in relation to fairness, see Broome 1991). Mooney (1998) suggests that there is a sub-set of claims—communitarian claims—which are the responsibility of the community to address. According to Mooney, 'The more embedded individuals are in a community and the greater the recognition of such embeddedness, the greater will be the strength of communitarian claims in that community'. In the context of a discussion about why we care about the health or welfare of others, the community—perhaps through its elected representatives—may decide that the worst-off individuals have a legitimate claim on those resources that will make them better off. Alternatively, the community may decide that those who have the highest capacity to benefit have the greatest claims.

An obvious question that arises here, is where does a communitarian claim come from? According to Mooney, the preferences of the community decide what constitutes a claim, and what the relative strengths of different claims are to be. Community preferences are those that are elicited from individuals in their role as citizens rather than as consumers. In a wider sense, communitarian writers have drawn our attention to the importance of historical traditions and social solidarity in the development of theories of justice. Indeed, communitarians would reject the notion that it is possible to construct one single theory of justice by which to judge every society. Rather, they view principles of justice as being pluralistic and regard what is due to individuals or groups as being dependent upon community-specific standards. In this way, it becomes possible to explain why Americans are more committed to free markets in health care than the British or Norwegians.

5.5 **Conclusion**

From the preceding discussion, it should be clear that we have no problem with the idea that it is 'rational' to care for others. Indeed, it is widely recognized that the human species has developed in the way it has precisely *because* of our concerns for one another—and, even Charles Darwin expected that 'virtuous habits will grow stronger, becoming perhaps fixed by inheritance'. There are of course limits to this altruism (the complete subordination of one's own needs to the needs of others is taking things too far) and much depends on reciprocity and the closeness of our relationships with others. However, our concerns for the health or well-being of other members of our community are central to discussions of how to distribute health care.

The textbook responses to 'market failures' is to *correct* those failures through indirect measures such as the price mechanism, or through public regulations. The rationale in markets, where the concept that 'you can't have it if you can't pay for it' is acceptable, is to get the market going in the most efficient way. In most countries, this concept is not acceptable in the context of health care. Public health care is distributed according to the concept that 'you can't have it if you don't *need* it'. As such, there is widespread political support for the socialist ideology of financing and distributing health care on the basis of 'from each according to ability, to each according to need'.

The failure of the demand side of the market for health care, then, is more fundamental than in other sectors. The issue is not one of correcting or adjusting the market, but one of replacing it. Citizens themselves have preferences for a distributive criterion that may be completely at odds with the market. This is important to bear in mind when we come to discuss the various approaches that exist for conducting economic evaluations in Chapter 7. In particular, we need to bear in mind the distributive criterion upon which a method is based. But first we must complete our discussion of why markets might fail and consider what measures might be taken to overcome, or at least mitigate, these failures. The next chapter considers issues relating to the financing and regulation of the supply side.

Suggested reading

On the economic rationale for the public sector, see Barr, N. (1993) *The economics of the welfare state*. London: Weidenfeld and Nicolson.

On altruism, see Zamagni, S. (ed.) (1995) *The economics of altruism*. Edward Elgar.

On fairness and equity, see Brosio, G. and Hochman, H. (ed.) (1998) *Economic justice*. Edward Elgar.

For a nice (and brief) insight into communitarianism, see Etzioni, A. (1996) A moderate communitarian proposal. *Political Theory*, 24, 155–71.

6

Providing health care: finance and regulation

The previous two chapters set out the arguments for government intervention in the distribution of health care. This chapter turns the focus towards the supply side and discusses some key issues on the financing and regulation of health care provision.

Market failures have implications for how a market should be regulated. The idea that an 'invisible hand' will take a market towards an efficient allocation of resources becomes untenable if that market is not capable of standing on its own two feet (that is, if it does not come close to satisfying the assumptions of perfect competition). *Uncertainty* about the incidence of illness, *asymmetric information* of various kinds between the providers and the users of health care, and *externalities* in consumption all mean that there is the need for extensive regulation of the provision of health care. Whilst private insurance markets can to some extent solve the problems associated with uncertainty, asymmetric information requires considerable government regulation to protect relatively uniformed users, and we have already seen that concerns for other people's health have implications for how health services should be financed.

An essential feature of most health services around the world is the constant pressure for more expenditure. The health policy challenge, then, is to impose regulatory measures on the providers of services so that total expenditures can be financed by the money that society is prepared to allocate for health care.

Much of what follows draws on the 'revenue–expenditure–income' identity of Bob Evans (for example, Evans 1997). We start with an inquiry into the possible sources for financing health care. This *revenue* would represent society's budget constraints for health care *expenditure*. This expenditure will always end up as *income* to those who provide the services. It is an indisputable fact that a given expenditure by one agent will always end up as a similarly sized income to one or more other agents.

6.1 **Flows of money: the 'revenue–expenditure–income' identity**

Revenues can be raised principally from four different sources: patient payments (*PP*), private insurance (*PI*), taxation for health (*TH*) (which also consolidates social insurance systems), and voluntary donations (*VD*). These in sum will represent the total budget for possible expenditure, which is determined by the unit cost (*C*) of the different health care commodities and the quantities (*Q*) of each. These, in turn, are produced by a combination of inputs, such as labour, capital, and raw materials, each of which are paid a unit rate. For simplicity, and without loss of generality, we can assume that everything ends up as labour income, as determined by the hours of labour (*L*) and the wage rate (*W*) per hour (which, of course, differ across the various professions involved).

More formally, the 'revenue–expenditure–income' identity can be expressed as in eqn 6.1, in which, for simplicity, the symbols refer to vectors:

$$
\begin{array}{ccccc}
\text{Revenues} & \equiv & \text{Expenditures} & \equiv & \text{Income} \\
PP + PI + TH + VD & \equiv & C * Q & \equiv & W * L.
\end{array}
\tag{6.1}
$$

The heart of the issue here is that the identity holds as a matter of logic and simple mathematical consistency. Any change in one parameter will initiate changes in at least one other parameter. It can either be offset or balanced by a change in other parameters on the same side of the identity, or the change will lead to the same-sized total changes on both of the other two sides. An example of the former type of change is when taxes as a source of revenue are reduced but compensated for by a corresponding increase in patient payments ($[-\Delta TH] = [+\Delta PP]$). An example of the latter is that no such compensation takes place on the revenue side, implying the same reduction in the other two sides of the identity, for example, reduced quantity of health care (*Q*) and fewer employees in the health sector (*L*), that is, $TH\downarrow \rightarrow Q\downarrow \rightarrow L\downarrow$. However, revenue reductions do not *imply* the same relative reductions in health care—labour productivity may improve, so that *C* falls rather than *Q*.

There are some important distinctions that can be made between the four sources of revenue. Patient payments come in many guises, such as deductibles (where the patient pays the first fixed amount of any costs) and charges (or cost-sharing, coinsurance, copayments, out-of-pocket payments—where the patient pays a given percentage of any costs). The characteristic feature of this source of funding is that it is levied after it has been established that the patient requires health care. Thus, there is a direct link between PP and $C*Q$.

The remaining sources of revenue would normally be paid prior to the possible need for health care. Private insurance premiums are—by definition—paid prior to an event, whereby an insurance holder is purchasing a guarantee of receipt of care (and attenuation of its cost), if needed. There is no cross-subsidization involved in private insurance, because the premium is based upon the expected losses of the insurance holder.

Taxation and voluntary donations differ from the other sources of revenue in that they involve *cross-subsidization*; that is, the rich or healthy subsidize the poor or sick. Income taxes are normally progressive, or at least proportionate, so high-income earners contribute more than low-income earners to the financing of public health care. Furthermore, when there is an inverse relationship between sickness and income, high-income groups also cross-subsidize low-income groups' use of health care. In other words, high-income earners *contribute more* than average to the funding of health care, and *use less* than average of the total services provided. Taxation differs from the above sources of funding in that it is compulsory. Also, income taxes may result in welfare losses in the labour market, given that the labour supply curve increases with income (more on this below).

Whilst the slice of total tax revenues that goes to public health care is a political decision in most countries, cross-subsidization is also an essential feature of publicly funded health care. Hence, tax-financed health care includes two analytically distinct elements; insurance for the tax-payer and their family and a cross-subsidization from those whose contributions exceed the costs of their own expected health care use to those whose contributions are less than their expected use. Voluntary donations include donations to health charities, as well as any direct financial support to hospitals and health care institutions in the community, and clearly represent cross-subsidized health care.

6.1.1 Limited revenue

There are limits to how much money people are willing to allocate towards their health care. First, when private health insurance is an option, there is a choice about which of the available packages to opt for. As with any other insurance purchase—be it car or house insurance, consumers make trade-offs between how much money to spend on this particular good compared with all other goods. There is an opportunity cost in the foregone benefits of expenditure on other things besides health insurance. Except perhaps for a few very rich people, most of us cannot afford an insurance policy that guarantees the immediate availability of all technologically feasible health care with the best amenities free of charge. Similarly, voluntary donations to the funding of other people's health care also have an upper limit, due to an opportunity cost in terms of less money for own private consumption. As such, we have a 'strained mercy'.

Clearly, when politicians decide how much of the total tax revenue should go to health care, they must recognize the opportunity costs in terms of the foregone benefits in other areas such as education, art, policing, and so on. Hence, politicians, as well as consumers, make trade-offs. The aggregated choices of consumers and politicians determine the total revenue that is made available for health care expenditure.

6.1.2 Keeping expenditures in line with revenues

Except for patient payments, the revenues available for producing health care are set at the start of the period under consideration. The challenge then is to keep expenditure within these constrained budgets. However, users and providers exert pressure. In the real world, advocates of *PP* rely almost entirely on the argument that publicly funded health care is 'underfunded' and needs private supplementation in order to satisfy 'unmet needs'. Beyond this underfunding argument, an efficiency argument is sometimes used—that *PP* will deter frivolous demand. This refers to health care with a small impact on health. However, because care seekers are not sufficiently informed to distinguish between effective and ineffective health care, copayments may result in a reduction in demand that is quite independent of the effectiveness of health care.

A consequence of reduced demand for health care is less *non-price rationing* in terms of waiting time. Of course this is fine for user groups with high time costs, who may then increase their demand. Hence, a distributive consequence of *PP* in relation to access to health care is that poor people are deterred (because they are more sensitive to the higher money costs) while rich people are attracted (because they are more sensitive to the lower time costs).

In general, health care is *not* demanded for its own sake, but for its expected positive outcomes. And because consumers have little information about the impact of health care on health (HC → H), they rely on the information and recommendations from providers of health care, for example, physicians or pharmaceutical companies. If providers consider themselves to be agents for the users, they will have a tendency to recommend all services that have positive expected outcomes. If providers strictly follow the ethical principle of *beneficience*, they will recommend the best possible treatments—regardless of costs. However, if the costs cannot be covered by society's budgets, policies are required for restricting the freedom providers have for making referrals to any kind of service with an expected positive outcome. Chapter 7 discusses the various economic evaluation methodologies that can be used to assist such policies.

6.1.3 Earning incomes from the expenditures

Doctors may well have an ethical justification for the excess provision of health care (excess in terms of going outside a given budget)—'the health of my patient shall be my first consideration'. However, there may also be financial incentives associated with excess provision—'the health care of my patient is my source of income'. Depending on the remuneration system, doctors' incomes may vary with the quantity (but not always with the quality) of services provided.

Other suppliers of services, such as the producers of pharmaceuticals and medical technology, have less ethical constraints than doctors who have face-to-face contacts with users. The objective function of these suppliers is more likely to be similar to that of other actors on the supply side in a normal market; namely, profit maximization. With this in mind, eqn 6.1 allows us to look at the impact of cost-containment policies which 'squeeze' these profits. For example, reductions in C^*Q imply similarly sized reductions in W^*L, so that wages will be cut or people will lose their jobs. Little wonder, then, that politicians have a hard time convincing groups who earn their incomes from health expenditures (such as doctors, lawyers, and pharmaceutical companies) of the merits of cost containment.

6.2 Disaggregation: a closer look at gainers and losers

Clearly, while the identity in eqn 6.1 holds in aggregate, it must be a very special case for the identity to hold for a particular individual. In eqn 6.2, we have indexed people by i, health care service by j, and factor input (labour) by k. In addition, p_j is the copayment for service j, q_{ij} is the quantity of j consumed by i, and c_j is the unit cost of producing j. Person i's private insurance, PI_i, might reflect an actuarially fair premium, but at least it is based upon i's expected insurance claims.

It is assumed that tax is paid at a proportional rate, t, with income, Y. The revenue side is made complete by having disaggregated voluntary donations, VD_i. The wage rate varies across professions, and the income earned by a person will consequently depend on their skills, w_k, and how many hours she works, L_{ik}.

$$\text{Revenues} \equiv \text{Expenditures} \equiv \text{Income} \quad (6.2)$$
$$\sum_i \left[\sum_j (p_j * q_{ij}) + PI_i + tY_i + VD_i \right] \equiv \sum_{ij}(c_j * q_{ij}) \equiv \sum_{ik}(w_k * L_{ik}).$$

First, let us abstract away those who earn their incomes from the production of health care services, and consider the revenue and expenditure sides only. An individual may contribute more than the costs of their health care use (revenues > expenditures) and is therefore a 'net loser'. Or she might contribute less than the costs of her health care (revenues < expenditures) and is therefore a 'net gainer' (at least in financial terms—in utility terms she might be classified a loser because she needs health care).

6.2.1 Shifting the financial burdens

Taxation and voluntary donations $(tY_i + VD_i)$ are based on the dictum 'from each according to his ability'. However, although an individual may have financial ability, they may still disapprove of contributing towards the care of others. Some groups of 'net losers' and their policy advocates seem to keep a constant pressure for shifting the financial burden. In most rich countries, voluntary donations to health care constitute only a small fraction of the total revenues, and rarely would we see political pressures against such donations. Still, when individuals choose to reduce their personal donations—which usually come from the wealthy and healthy—this implies that compulsory taxes will have to increase, or that patients will have to pay higher charges.

A given reduction in tax financing implies that patient payments increase, or that citizens go for private health insurance. By definition, increased patient payments shift the financial burden towards patients. Private insurance financing is regressive for two reasons. First, the premium is set *independent of income*, so the lower one's income, the higher is the share of income paid for a given amount of coverage. Second, to the extent that illness—and thus the expected need for health care resources—is negatively correlated with income, the actuarially fair premiums for low-income earners would consequently be *higher* than for high-income earners. Hence, shifting the financial burden from taxation to patient payments and private insurance implies a similar shift in the principle for distributing health care: rather than 'to each according to their needs', it implies 'to each according to their ability to pay'.

6.2.2 Making a living from expenditure

Popular policies do not come free. Wage increases for health care personnel are popular—at least amongst health care personnel. If there is no reduction in the total hours worked or in the number of employees, this will increase total expenditure—for which revenues have to be sought in one of the four alternative ways indicated in Section 6.1. Reduced patient payments are also popular—at least amongst patients. If the other sources of revenue do not offset reduced patient payments, then there will be less expenditure on health care, and consequently lower total incomes for health care personnel and the whole range of service contractors.

The incomes of most health care personnel depend on their wage rate and the hours worked. However, physicians' incomes may also depend on the quantity and type of services provided, or the size of their patient lists. The ways in which incomes and remuneration systems affect provider behaviour is indeed a huge topic in health economics—sufficient for a book in itself. In this book we shall briefly consider some key aspects, and will start with the 'public–private mix'.

6.3 The split between purchasers and providers

First, consider Fig. 6.1 that comes from the field of public economics and illustrates the important distinction between finance and provision when discussing the public–private mix (for simplicity we have abstracted away voluntary donations). How should the particular service be financed (public or private)? What is the most efficient way of providing the service (public or private)?

The vertical choice is essentially a normative one. It depends on the policy objectives regarding the principles upon which health care should be distributed. If this is 'equal access independent of income', there is a strong case against private finance. However, for the types of services for which it is accepted that access could depend on income, society might accept to move to the right of the vertical bold line of Fig. 6.1.

| | | Finance | |
		Public	Private
Provision	Public	1	2
	Private	3	4

Fig. 6.1 The public–private mix in finance and provision.

The horizontal choice is more about finding the best 'means to an end'. It crucially depends on which types of ownership, organization, and regulation will produce services of specified qualities in the least costly way. There are strong political views and traditions here, where 'leftists' tend to believe that the public sector is better able to provide quality services at low cost, and 'rightists' tend to believe that the private sector is best. However, having decided on the *normative* issue (how the services should be financed), the question on who is the best to provide them is essentially a *positive* one.

Political discussions of the various attempts to privatize a public health service can be set within the framework of Fig. 6.1. They deal either with the privatization of finance (a horizontal move from box 1 to box 2) or with the privatization of provision (a vertical move from box 1 to box 3). The former has either a political rationale ('the government cannot afford more expenses') or it has the welfare economic rationale of reducing the so-called welfare loss from taxation. Vertical privatization involves a range of terms—'outsourcing', 'opting-out', 'competition', and so on—all of which *should* be motivated by expected increases in efficiency.

Once the money has been channelled to purchasers (such as general practitioners (GPs)), the question becomes how the money flows from the purchasers to the providers (such as hospitals), that is, the ways in which providers are reimbursed for their services. Figure 6.2 represents the grand picture of the money and resource flows between the three parts; households (citizens and patients); purchasers (government and private insurance as 'third-party payers'); and providers (primary and secondary care). Households pay for health care, directly through patient payments or voluntary donations, and indirectly in terms of taxes and private insurance. Health care providers are paid directly in terms of patient payments from patients and voluntary donations from households, or indirectly in terms

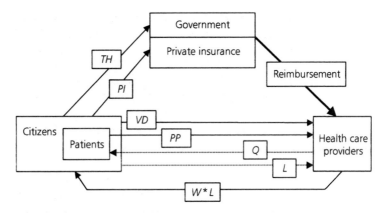

Fig. 6.2 The money flows in health care finance and provision. See text for explanation and definitions of abbreviations.

of reimbursements from the third party. The resources required for producing health care are the labour inputs delivered from the households, for which incomes ($W*L$) are paid in return. In addition to the money flows, there are service and resource flows illustrated by the dotted arrows. Patients receive health care (Q) from health care providers, and households deliver the resources required for producing these services, which has been simplified to consist of labour input only (L).

Figure 6.2 reflects eqn 6.1 in that the total revenues ($TH + PI + VD + PP$) equal expenditures ($C*Q$), which again equal incomes ($W*L$). However, this figure highlights something hidden in the equation; namely, the money flows that pass via the third-party payers, and the range of ways that the third parties could possibly reimburse those who provide health care. Reimbursement policies are a central part of health policy. First, by logic, there is no more money to be reimbursed than the money made available through the third-party payers in terms of taxes and insurance. If providers want more health care, they have to raise funding from patient payments or voluntary donations. Second, reimbursement mechanisms impact upon which services are provided to which patient groups. As such, reimbursement policies influence *provider behaviour*.

The pressure for more health care than the sum of $TH + PI$ arises from the (un)holy alliance between patients and providers. If doctors consider themselves to be *agents for patients* in that they would respond to the wishes of their patients, then the total costs of the preferred level of care are likely to exceed the revenues available. However, if doctors were to consider themselves as *agents for society* (or for third-party payers), they would be conscious not to use more resources than the budgets allow for. As alluded to in Section 4.5, this dual agency role means that doctors are pulled in different directions. Patients as consumers might threaten to sue doctors who do not provide what they want. Purchasers might say 'you can't always get what you want'—and patients as citizens might acknowledge that 'we can't always get what we want'—and seek to design reimbursement systems that make providers meet their (that is, purchasers or patients as citizens) objectives.

Except for acute and emergency admissions, in most health care systems potential patients seek *primary care* first. At this level, GPs or family doctors make decisions about whether to refer a patient on to *secondary care* (that is, specialists and hospitals). A critical policy issue for the third-party payer is whether to let *internal markets* operate between primary and secondary care. In the absence of such markets, GPs refer their patients to hospitals and trust that the specialists will recognize their patient's needs and treat them. But since GPs face no costs in referring their patients to hospitals, they have no financial reason to modify their demand for secondary care. Consequently, excess demand ensues. However, in the presence of internal markets, GPs do not have to cross their own—nor their patients— fingers. Rather, if they feel that their patient's needs for specialist treatment are convincing enough, then they can use their budgets to buy secondary care for those patients.

Internal markets were introduced in the UK in the 1980s under the Conservative government who were keen to reduce costs in the National Health Service (NHS) and public services generally. The separation of the provision and financing of health care was to be achieved by allowing hospitals to become self-governing 'NHS Trusts', whereby they would contract with 'District General Managers' and 'GP fundholders'. In theory, all hospitals would compete with one another to provide services to purchasers. Thus, money 'follows the patient' to wherever the best care can be acquired most efficiently. To facilitate competition, trusts were to have greater control over their assets and revenues. Detailed contracts would be used to specify the relationship between purchasers and providers. The internal market was reinforced by giving larger GP practices the option of controlling their own budgets and many of these chose to become GP fundholders. Again through the use of detailed contracts, the aim was to encourage the audit of activity and costs.

On efficiency issues, many of the reforms were welcomed by health economists, but change took place far too quickly to allow careful evaluation of their effects. With regard to equity, the encouragement of the private sector called into question whether 'the NHS is safe in their hands'. The election of the Labour government in 1997 saw the retention of the purchaser–provider split and an increased emphasis on a primary care-led NHS. However, in a partial rejection of the internal market, short-term contracts (with all their associated transaction costs) were replaced with long-term agreements. In addition, GP fundholding was withdrawn because patients of fundholders were being treated before patients of non-fundholding GPs, and replaced by primary care groups (groups of GP practices) who contracted with hospitals. The questions here have been about who holds which budgets. But irrespective of the sources of revenue for hospitals (be it third-party payer, patients, or GPs), a common problem is how to get their employees to work more in response to increased demand for their services, and thus we need to consider the supply of labour.

6.4 **Labour supply**

The most important input factor in the production of health care is labour. Thus, in order to provide more health care, more labour is required. While there are many things that affect an individual's choice of how much to work, the wage rate is certainly a crucial variable and therefore an important incentive device. In general, the higher the wage rate of a profession, the more people who possess the particular skills will prefer to work. For example, the higher the annual wage of nurses, then more of those qualified will prefer to work as a nurse rather than stay at home or choose other professions. And in the long run, the higher the wage rate of a profession, the more people will be attracted to attain the required skills.

As to the choice of *how much* to work, the conventional perception seems to be that the same causal relation exists as for the choice of *whether* to work, namely that increases in the wage rate will always attract a person to work more. However, this is not necessarily the case, and we will explain why within the context of a general model on labour supply.

Consider an individual who faces a time constraint. During a given time period (a year, a week, or a day), a given proportion is devoted to work, and the rest is leisure (even if it is spent doing household chores). The income an individual receives depends on how much they work and the wage rate. In what follows, we will assume that all other things that may affect labour supply are constant and that the only relevant 'goodies' in life are income (from which consumption goods can be purchased) and leisure.

By implication, it follows that work is 'a bad' that has instrumental value only—in terms of it being a source of income (this is unfortunately true for many people, though not all).

Now consider the situation where an individual can freely choose the number of hours worked. Except for the variables on the axes, Fig. 6.3 is similar to Fig. 2.6 in that it illustrates an indifference curve, U_0, a budget constraint, and the optimal choice at point A, given the constraint (a more realistic budget line would account for a minimum wage, or supplementary benefits if out of work, as well as a minimum leisure time required for sleeping). The horizontal axis measures the number of hours for leisure, H_L, which has a logical maximum (only 24 h in a day) at the intersection, H_L^{max}. The vertical axis measures income, I, with a maximum income— shown at I^{max} (!) The slope of the budget line is the wage rate, w_0. Given the wage rate and the leisure–income preferences of this individual, their demand for leisure is shown by H_L^0 and their corresponding supply of labour, or working hours, becomes $H_W^0 = (H_L^{max} - H_L^0)$, yielding an income of $I_0 = w_0 * H_W^0$.

Then what happens with an increase in the wage rate? Figure 6.4 illustrates this by a steeper budget line. The individual can move further out in their utility space and land at a point C where an indifference curve, U_1, is tangential to the new budget line. There are two simultaneous effects taking place now. First, there is an *income effect* that follows from the fact that leisure is a 'normal good' (defined as a good for which an individual would increase their demand when their income increases), that is, the higher

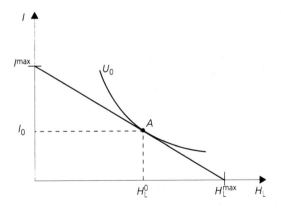

Fig. 6.3 The preferred combination of income and leisure.

their income, the more leisure they can afford, and thus the more they will demand. In isolation, this partial effect of a wage increase would imply a *reduced* supply of labour. Second, there is a *substitution effect* that follows from the fact that leisure has become more expensive, in that the foregone income from *not* working an extra hour is higher, that is, the opportunity costs of leisure have increased. This partial effect of leisure having become a more expensive good would imply less demand for it with a corresponding *increased supply* of labour.

In Fig. 6.4, we have illustrated the two partial effects by adding a hypothetical budget line that is parallel to the new budget line and tangential to the initial indifference curve at point *B*. This point is characterized by leaving the individual at their initial utility level but with the new wage rate. A real world policy that might explain this hypothetical shift would be the introduction of a poll tax and a wage increase which make the individual as happy as before, that is, they are indifferent between *A* and *B*. However, at this new point they work more *and* get a higher income (higher than the poll tax). When this hypothetical poll tax is abolished, they move from *B* to *C*, a move that is characterized by more leisure and more income. In other words, the result of the wage increase can then be explained by a substitution effect from *A* to *B* and an income effect from *B* to *C*. Given that these two effects work in opposite directions with regard to labour supply, the question is which effect is larger in absolute terms? Figure 6.4 has illustrated a situation with *increased* labour supply, but it is easy to draw an indifference curve whereby labour supply *decreases*.

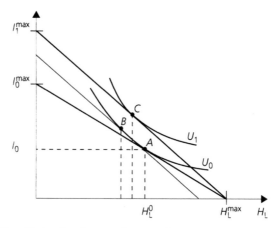

Fig. 6.4 The effects of an increased wage rate.

By making further increases in the wage rate, the loci of the preferred income–leisure points can be identified. These points can then be translated into a *supply curve* for labour in Fig. 6.5, where the horizontal axis measures the number of working hours, H_W, and the vertical axis measures the wage rate, w. We have illustrated a backward bending curve, whereby increases in the wage rate will lead to increased labour supply if the wage is low, but will lead to reduced labour supply when the wage rates become very high.

This shape of the labour supply curve is often found in economics textbooks. However, the point at which the curve starts to bend backwards is far from clear cut. The empirical evidence is mixed and economists naturally disagree on this. Still, this model may help to explain how health care personnel respond to changes in their wage systems. First, tax increases (which imply corresponding reductions in the wage rate) may result in *increased* labour supply for those individuals located at the backward bending part of the curve. This is contrary to the conventional wisdom that income taxes always have negative incentives on labour supply. (Interestingly, this is also contrary to the 'welfare loss' argument against income taxation in general and against tax-financed health care in particular.) There is also evidence that people respond to reductions in the wage rate by increasing the labour supply in order to maintain a given income level. In the health economics literature, such behaviour is referred to as reflecting the 'target income hypothesis' (remember the study by

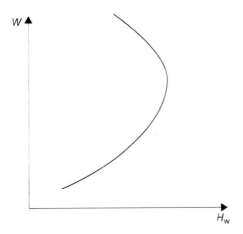

Fig. 6.5 The labour supply curve.

Krasnik *et al.* discussed under the topic of supplier-induced demand in Chapter 4).

Second, the above figure is based on the premise that wage rates are determined exogenously, and that individuals adjust their supply of labour in accordance with their leisure–income preferences. Under some remuneration systems, physicians may have discretion to influence their implicit wage rate depending on their style of practice. Under 'fee-for-service' systems, the more services they prescribe per hour, the higher the implicit wage rate. Under 'capitation' systems, the shorter the consultation for each patient, the more patients on the list, and—again—the higher the implicit wage rate.

Third, one lesson from the framework of Figs 6.3 and 6.4 is that it is the *marginal* wage rate that influences a person's propensity to supply an additional hour of their labour. So, when comparing a high base rate independently of how many hours are worked against a system with a low base rate for normal hours and increasingly high overtime rates, this latter wage package will generate a higher supply of labour. Thus, if skilled health care personnel is scarce and hospitals want their employees to increase their labour supply, it would be better to design a wage system with increasing overtime rates than to increase the base rate. The alternative, with an increased base rate, means that *income effect* becomes relatively large, and so there is the danger of hitting the backward bending part of the labour supply curve. However, incentives which are successful in terms of making health care personnel work long hours are not necessarily compatible with making happy families. Since this is a topic that certainly lies outside the scope of this book, we leave it here.

6.5 **Conclusion**

The founder of the British NHS, Aneurin Bevan, said that 'if you want to send a message to a doctor, you must write it on a cheque'. But often people behave in ways we expect them to. So, if we design a sophisticated payment system in which one's income depends on 'every move you make, every step you take', doctors may easily end up with a selfish pecuniary eye on every clinical decision. Alternative incentives lie in appealing to other aspects of doctors' practices that are important to them, such as professional ethics, and competence and qualifications; that is, being a good doctor both morally and technically.

While doctor bashing is popular amongst economists, we do not believe that doctors—a priori—are any worse than other professions with the same length of education (or status). Still, we pause to wonder why there is so much variety in the wage systems of doctors, where each system is judged according to how effective its financial incentives are in making doctors act in accordance with stated policy objectives. Most other public-sector professionals are salaried and are assumed not to need any additional financial incentives to make them work appropriately.

This book is not a moral manifesto to doctors, and we leave it to others to suggest how professional ethics may help us get even better doctors than we already have. In helping doctors choose the best treatment among the alternative options, increasing use is made of 'evidence-based medicine', 'health-technology assessments', and 'clinical guidelines'. All of these represent attempts at reducing ineffective procedures and interventions and, at some level, require the comparison of expected health outcomes with costs. We now turn to a discussion of the methodologies that can be used to compare what you get with what you have to pay for it.

Suggested reading

On the 'revenue–expenditure–income' identity, see Evans, R. G. (1997) Going for the gold: the redistributive agenda behind market-based health care reforms. *Journal of Health Politics, Policy and Law*, 22, 427–65.

On the public–private mix, see Stiglitz, J. (1988) *Economics of the public sector*. Norton, New York.

On labour supply, see the suggested reading in Chapter 2.

7

Economic evaluation techniques

Economic evaluations seek to aid the comparison of alternative treatments within and across programme areas. This chapter discusses some of the different economic evaluation techniques, and focuses on the normative issues associated with their use in informing resource-allocation decisions.

The various economic evaluation techniques focus on those attributes of health care programmes that can be classified as costs and benefits. Clearly, if there are no expected benefits from a programme, there is no point in providing it (hopefully nobody would disagree with us on this). The importance of costs is obvious to economists. Resources are scarce, and they will therefore always have an alternative use. The so-called 'opportunity costs' refer to the 'benefits foregone' from the best alternative use of the resources spent. What seems to be less obvious to economists, though, is to understand why in some situations people would neglect the relevance of cost differences—something that will be discussed in Chapter 8. Also in Chapter 8, we will discuss other relevant aspects beyond those that can be squeezed in under the headings of costs or benefits.

7.1 Different techniques with some basic similarities

Controversies exist in the literature as to which economic evaluation methodology is the best—or 'the theoretically most correct'. Students sometimes get the impression that the different camps each have a preferred approach, independent of the specific policy question. To us, the appropriate method to use crucially depends on the question being asked, as well as on the value basis of the institution whose decision making the evaluation is meant to assist. There are essentially two types of questions. The first asks which of two (or more) alternative treatments for the *same* type of condition is preferred? The second asks which of two (or more) alternative treatments for *different* types of condition is preferred? In other words, we face choices about how best to choose between treatments within the same condition (that is, technical efficiency) and across different conditions (that is, allocative efficiency). Comparisons that address allocative efficiency become meaningful only when the different dimensions of benefit have been translated into a common currency, so that they become *commensurable*.

The ways in which benefits are being measured appears to be the distinguishing feature of the various economic evaluation techniques—tell us in which ways the benefits have been measured and we will give you the label for the method used. Table 7.1 distinguishes the methods depending on whether benefits have been measured in monetary terms or not and whether benefits are based on preferences or not. When benefits are measured in money, they—by definition—become comparable to costs. An economic evaluation in which benefits are measured in monetary terms is referred to as a cost–benefit analysis (CBA). However, economists often reserve the CBA label for those analyses that have their theoretical basis in neo-classical welfare economics. Here, benefits are based on preferences that reflect the consumers' valuations, for example, as expressed through their willingness to pay. Although many economists might not use the label CBA if benefits are *not* based on preferences, non-economists might. Furthermore, a 'welfare economic CBA' is not necessarily more policy relevant than a CBA in which benefits are measured in other ways (see Section 7.2.1 below).

If benefits are *not* measured in monetary terms, some sort of cost-effectiveness analysis (CEA) is used. An important group of CEA in the health economics literature is what has come to be labelled 'cost–utility analysis' (CUA). The use of the word 'utility' here is because the benefit measure is claimed to be some measure of individual utility (from health).

Table 7.1 A taxonomy of economic evaluation technique

Benefits based on preferences	Benefits measured in monetary terms	
	Yes	**No**
Yes	CBA	CEA (CUA)
No	CBA (but *not* based on welfare economics)	CEA

CBA, cost–benefit analysis; CEA, cost-effectiveness analysis; CUA, cost–utility analysis.

In this table, the vertical distinction is clear cut in that benefits are either measured in monetary terms or they are not. If not, some units of health are normally used. The horizontal distinction separates out those techniques that do not have *any* bases in preferences. Among those techniques that do attempt to measure preferences, there is a wide range of possible sources of value, from those evaluations that make only very rough estimates of the utility from a health state to those which proclaim that preferences over all attributes of a programme have been assessed. The various ways in which preferences can be measured will be returned to later in this chapter.

For now consider the most general representation of what the various economic evaluation techniques have in common; namely, the comparison of costs and benefits. A programme evaluation starts out by *identifying* and *quantifying* (in physical units) the affected items and then categorizes them into being benefit items, indexed by i (B_i) or cost items, indexed by j (C_j). Costs are *valued* in money terms (V_j). Benefits (V_i) can be valued in three different ways: in monetary terms, in non-monetary terms, such as quality-of-life indices, or in physical or natural units, that is, 'in themselves', such as lives saved. Since benefits and costs occur at different points in time (t), a discount rate, r, is used to adjust for such time differences.

The policy question to which an economic evaluation is intended to provide an answer is whether the programme is worth pursuing. In economic terms, this is essentially the *potential Pareto criterion*, which looks at whether the gainers can potentially compensate the losers, that is, is the value to the beneficiaries larger than the losses to those who bear the costs? And, in cost–benefit terms, is the present value of the future stream of benefits greater than the future stream of costs? Using the symbols suggested above, this net present value (NPV), can be specified as in eqn 7.1:

$$\text{NPV} = \frac{\sum_t \sum_i (V_{it} \star B_{it})}{\sum_t (1 + r)^t} - \frac{\sum_t \sum_j (V_{jt} \star C_{jt})}{\sum_t (1 + r)^t}. \tag{7.1}$$

If this NPV calculation is greater than zero, then the programme is worth pursuing; if it is less than zero, then the programme is not worth pursuing.

Clearly, for the most general formula 7.1 to make sense, the first term must be measured in the same unit as the second, that is, benefits must be valued in monetary terms. Hence, eqn 7.1 refers—by definition—to CBA (see Table 7.1).

However, in the same way as apples and oranges cannot be added, apples cannot be *subtracted* from oranges (or vice versa). So, when we decide to value benefits in health terms, the first term of eqn 7.1 is being expressed in a different unit from the second term, and the formula becomes meaningless. In order to compare costs and benefits, eqn 7.1 is rearranged to become a ratio. The non-monetarized benefits in the denominator are referred to as *effects*, and so eqn 7.2 is the formula behind the cost-effectiveness ratio (CER):

$$CER = \frac{\sum_t \sum_j (V_{jt} * C_{jt})/\sum_t (1 + r)^t}{\sum_t \sum_i (V_{it} * B_{it})/\sum_t (1 + r)^t}. \tag{7.2}$$

This ratio does not in itself offer any policy-relevant information. It is only when compared with the ratios from alternative programmes that a new programme's relative goodness can be assessed.

The remainder of this chapter deals with each of the parameters in the above formulae. The following section discusses the various methods for valuing benefits in monetary units, that is, the V_{it} in formula 7.1. Section 7.3 goes on to deal with the valuation of benefits in *health* units. Section 7.4 discusses key principles in the estimation of costs. The final parameter (r) on time-adjustments is discussed in Section 7.5.

7.2 Valuing benefits in monetary terms

7.2.1 Non-preference-based measures of monetary benefits

The simplest way of measuring monetary benefits is through the narrow perspective of cost savings elsewhere. Will a health care programme lead to cost savings in the health sector or in other sectors of the economy?

It is sometimes used as an argument for prevention programmes that they are 'profitable' for the health sector, in that the reduced illnesses attributable to prevention imply reduced future treatment costs. In the framework of formula 7.1 the second term refers to the costs of a preventive programme while the first term refers to the present value of the future health care cost savings. It seems evident that if the net health sector costs are negative (and that no costs are imposed on other sectors), the programme should be implemented. However, for most programmes, net health care costs are positive, and so benefits would have to be found on other fronts in order to justify the costs. A broader perspective is to look for cost savings in other sectors of the economy as well. If these cost savings exceed the health care costs then—from the perspective of a societal economic evaluation—the programme should be implemented. Note that if costs are negative, the size of the health outcomes do not matter—as long as they are positive.

Returning again to Fig. 1.1 in Chapter 1, improved health may have positive effects on wealth. When sick workers are cured, society benefits in terms of the increased production that is attributable to their return to work. The appropriate method for measuring such effects has been a recurring theme in the economic evaluation literature. However, there are also conceptual confusions in this literature, due to misleading definitions as well as a tendency to apply a terminology from the cost-of-illness (COI) literature in the context of CEA. Cost of illness has a completely different perspective from CEA. In COI, the focus is the illness and the aim is to estimate the total costs to society of the illness—sometimes referred to as the economic 'burden of disease'. In CEA the focus of attention is *not the illness, but the intervention.*

There has been a terminological convention in the literature on economic evaluation to refer to direct versus indirect costs and benefits, of which the indirect benefits are the production gains *caused by the intervention*. The concepts used in COI and CEA have different meanings; 'indirect costs' in COI are 'indirect benefits' (averted production losses) in CEA. The distinction between 'direct' and 'indirect' is not particularly meaningful, as it depends on the institutional viewpoint of the analyses. With the viewpoint of an individual in Fig. 1.1., health *per se* has a direct benefit, but also an indirect benefit via the wealth created. As such, this distinction has some explanatory value. However, from the viewpoint of an employer who is concerned with the productivity of their input factors, production gains would be the *direct* benefit, while the benefit from improved health *per se*, as experienced by their labour, would be an *indirect* benefit. Thus, conceptual clarifications are required (see Olsen and Richardson 1999).

We shall use the term health care costs (HC) to refer to what the CEA literature sometimes terms *direct costs*. *Indirect costs* refer to all sorts of non-health care costs that accompany the treatment. Often these are measured as different types of time costs, the largest item of which is the production lost whilst undergoing treatment. Rather than indirect costs, we shall use the term production losses (PL). *Direct benefits* are health effects or health gains, which in CEA are non-monetarized health (H). *Indirect benefits* are, in the words used in the seminal paper by Torrance (1986) 'the production gains to society because more people are well, or alive, and able to return to work'. Thus, we prefer the term production gains (*PG*) for the value of the increased output that is attributable to the treatment.

Within a CBA, benefits are measured as increased production and become the first term of the general formula 7.1. The NPV then, becomes the production gains (*PG*) minus the programme costs (*HC* + *PL*):

$$NPV = PG - (HC + PL). \tag{7.3}$$

Clearly, if the mission of the analyst is to offer an economic argument in support of the programme, the higher the production gains, the better it appears for society. Note that benefits from improved health *per se* are not included in this type of CBA.

Within a CEA, the monetarized *PG* cannot appear in the denominator together with *non*-monetarized units of health, because incommensurable units cannot be added. Thus, *PG* have to appear in the numerator like a cost-saving to be subtracted in order to arrive at the 'net economic costs to society'. These costs are then divided by the number of health benefit units in order to derive a CER for health (eqn 7.4):

$$CER = \frac{(HC + PL) - PG}{H}. \tag{7.4}$$

If the denominator in eqn 7.4 were to include a preference-based attribute (for example, the *Q* for health-related quality of life), the formula would be termed a cost–utility ratio (more on this in Section 7.3.2 below).

Measuring benefits from health care in terms of production gains raises technical as well as normative questions. The former relate to what the correct approach to estimating the magnitude of these gains is. There are essentially two different methods for measuring *PG*, termed human capital and friction cost. With gross earnings as a proxy for the value of one's output, the present value of the future stream of earnings becomes one way of measuring the production gain to society of a person's return to work. The *human capital* approach uses averted lost earnings to estimate production gains.

The *friction cost* approach is different in that the focus lies on productivity changes rather than earnings. In economies with high unemployment, sick employees can eventually be replaced from the unemployment pool. The (avoided) lost output in this case would depend upon the reduced productivity of each of the people affected and the length of time before productivity returned to normal. In these circumstances, the lost output to society will be temporary, that is, it is limited to a *friction period*. The friction cost method, then, represents a technical response to the exaggerated estimates of lost output measured by the human capital method (Koopmanschap *et al.* 1995).

When the purpose is that of estimating the impact of a health care programme on society's production level, the idea behind the friction cost method seems the most correct. The human capital method would be correct if the purpose were that of estimating the earnings generated by previously sick and unproductive employees as a consequence of their return to work. The two methods would give similar results if income reflects the value of production, and if the employee were completely irreplaceable in the labour market. While the first assumption is a useful simplification, the second one is not realistic ('cemeteries are full of irreplaceable men').

Unfortunately, there is much confusion in some parts of the economic evaluation literature about which available figures should be used for assessing the economic benefits to society of a person's return to work. Some authors use gross income, some use net income, while others consider the government's savings of sickness benefits; there are even examples of adding 'debit and credit' (for example, income + sickness benefits). In attempting to clarify matters, we shall distinguish between the *real changes* in the value of society's production and *transfer payments* across different agents in the economy. Table 7.2 illustrates what happens when a previously sick worker returns to work. Consider the three parties: the worker, the employer, and the government. The employer experiences a production gain (PG)—attributable to the return of the worker, but has to pay a wage, W. The worker receives a net wage after taxation, T, but loses sickness benefits, SB. The government receives taxation and gains from not having to pay sickness benefits. In this case, the government acts as a social insurer, but the principle point of transfer payments would hold under private insurance schemes as

Table 7.2 The return of a productive worker: real production effects versus transfers

	Worker	Employer	Government
Increased production		$+PG$	
Wage impacts	$+(W - T)$	$-W$	$+T$
Sickness benefits	$-SB$		$+SB$

PG, production gain; *W*, wage; *T*, taxation; *SB*, sickness benefits.

well. Table 7.2 illustrates how transfers are being 'netted out' across the three parties. Thus, what remains is what matters; namely, the production gains.

Beyond this positive issue of correctly assessing the magnitude of production gains, there is the normative issue of how much of such gains should be accounted for in a societal economic analysis. The higher production gains that follow from the treatment of a particular patient group, the more is being subtracted in the numerator of eqn 7.4, and hence the more favourable the ratio becomes. Thus, priority is given to the most productive in society at the expense of groups who—for various reasons—are less productive. This explains why some authors object to including *PG*. A closer look at where production gains may end up suggests that gains in terms of private consumption are not necessarily something that society would wish to subtract in the numerator of eqn 7.4. Interestingly, the US panel that discussed guidelines for CEA argued for taking account of 'only the impact on the *rest* of society' (Weinstein *et al.* 1997). So, the panel suggested that taxes and voluntary contributions to the rest of society represent the types of gains relevant in a CEA (an elaboration of the arguments for such restricted inclusion of production gains can be found in Olsen and Richardson 1999).

7.2.2 Preference-based measures of monetary benefits

There is a saying that 'economists have preferences, psychologists have attitudes'. More accurately, economists believe that *consumers* have preferences, and that these preferences can be *revealed* from actual behaviour in markets, where trade-offs are made across different goods with different attributes. Alternatively, consumers can *state* their preferences through choices presented to them in hypothetical questions.

In general, economists have a preference for revealed preferences, because they put more faith in how people *actually* behave than in how people *say* they would behave. This principle is fine in situations where markets provide the goods but when the goods that we want to value are not available in ordinary markets, preferences have to be elicited in other ways. Preferences for health could in principle be revealed from actual behaviour but in contrast to 'normal market goods' there are relatively few situations in which people can reveal implicit monetary values for the health improvement that health care might provide. Rarely do we find market analogues through which consumers have had the opportunity to signal their values of health improvements.

Moreover, the market for health care is characterized by so many failures (see Chapter 4) that it is exceedingly difficult to infer consumers' precise valuations of particular health interventions. First, rarely do health care consumers have experience from previous purchases (fortunately, most surgeries are a once-in-a-life-time experience). Second, they lack information about the qualities of the goods to be able to assess an expected monetary value. Third, there are so many probability terms involved that few people are able to rationally calculate their subjective value of a particular treatment (assuming that a private insurance option exists for this treatment).

The value of safety appears to occupy a middle ground between 'normal goods' and health regarding the feasibility of inferring consumers' monetary values from revealed behaviour. A range of safety features are available in the market (for example, safe cars and smoke detectors), and by dividing the price of a safety feature with its marginal risk reduction, an *implicit value of life* can be inferred. Comparisons of such estimates of implicit values of life show huge variations across different types of risk-reducing goods (see Tengs *et al.* 1995). Thus, notwithstanding market failures, consumers are either misinformed about the magnitude of various risk reductions or they have very clear views on how they would prefer *not* to die.

For goods that are not available in well-functioning markets, economists have developed methods for constructing hypothetical markets. These methods are termed *contingent valuation*, whereby respondents are asked to express a value that would be true under certain specified conditions. Contingent valuation is an umbrella term for different types of hypothetical monetary evaluation questions, each of which would be associated with a specific theoretical utility measure (see a standard micro-economic textbook, and look for 'compensating variation' and 'equivalent variation'). By far the most widely applied version of contingent valuation in health and health care is the willingness-to-pay (WTP) method.

WTP has—like other contingent valuation methods—its theoretical basis in neo-classical welfare economics. It is founded on the dictum that a good has *value* to a consumer only to the extent that they are prepared to *sacrifice* something in order to obtain it. So, the more they are willing to sacrifice of their own income, the higher is the value of the good in question. The maximum WTP would then express the respondent's valuation of the good in monetary terms. A crucial assumption here is that more is better (at least up to a meaningful satiation level), that is, the larger the quantity of the particular good, the more income they are prepared to sacrifice for it.

The logical starting point in a WTP study is to specify what exactly is being valued. A key concept here is the *scenario description* that explains the characteristics of the particular good. For health care, it is important to describe types of outcomes, as well as the process of treatment if that is considered relevant. Ideally, information on all the assumed utility- (and disutility-) yielding attributes of the programme should be provided. However, the cognitive capacity of respondents obviously represents a constraint on how much information can be dealt with.

A second issue, and one that has attracted much interest, is the question format, that is, how the WTP question should be phrased. There are four alternatives: (1) *open-ended*, which basically asks 'how much would you be willing to pay?' without giving any reference sum; (2) *closed ended*, which asks 'would you be willing to pay X dollars?', where X is varied across sub-samples, and a demand curve is estimated based on how the fraction of yes-respondents varies across sub-samples; (3) *iterative bidding games*, whereby the interviewer starts with a specified bid, and follows up by asking if higher or lower sums would be acceptable depending on the answer to the preceding bid; and (4) *payment cards*, where alternative sums are listed, usually from zero to a realistic maximum, and where respondents are asked to circle the amount which comes closest to their maximum WTP. In this literature, there are different camps holding fairly strong views on which question format is the best—or most correct. However, the scientific attention to this methodological issue does not seem to correspond with its applied importance in terms of the relative differences in mean values that the methods seem to produce.

In fact, there are other problems with WTP that are more severe in terms of the reliability of responses. Beattie *et al.* (1998) suggested that WTP answers are 'sensitive to theoretically *ir*relevant factors, and *in*sensitive to theoretically relevant factors'. Probably the most important *relevant* factor is the size of the good—people should be willing to pay more for more. But there is much evidence that WTP is insensitive to the magnitude of such things as the size of the risk reductions and the scope of the environmental benefit. And there is now some supporting evidence from the health field, which shows that WTP is insensitive to the size of health outcomes (Olsen *et al.* 2001). In fact, *within*-respondent tests in this study showed that the majority of respondents do not increase their WTP for the programme when the size of the outcome doubles. Clearly, rational individuals would agree that if a programme A treats twice the number of patients as programme B, then A is better for society than B. But the valuation instrument does not pick this up, and so the validity of this instrument is called into question.

Examples of theoretically *ir*relevant factors include the fact that slight changes in the wording of scenario descriptions can have dramatic effects on stated WTP and the finding that the respondent's valuation of a preceding programme can affect their value of a subsequent programme. When the most significant determinant of a respondent's WTP for programme B is their WTP for a previously valued (and completely different) programme A, their valuation cannot be 'independent of irrelevant alternatives', and doubt must again be cast on the reliability of WTP responses.

Of the methods that exist for measuring benefits from health care in monetary terms, economists tend to favour preference-based measures because of their theoretical appeal. However, the recent evidence of measurement problems from applied studies seems to have increased the level of scepticism, and the theoretically preferred alternative is not necessarily the most reliable in practice.

7.3 Valuing benefits in health terms

7.3.1 Non-preference-based health benefits

Survival rates have been a widely used outcome measure in health. An intervention is counted as a success if patients survive for five years, say— and as a failure if they do not. This is obviously a very crude measure, because it does not distinguish between having survived 1 week or 4.9 years, or between surviving 5 years or 50 years. An alternative, therefore, is to count life years, so that the numeraire is no longer persons but years.

The good thing with survival rates and life years is that they are commensurate terms for mortality, thus facilitating comparisons across programme areas. The bad thing, however, is that they neglect differences in morbidity. There now exists a wide range of outcome measures for improved morbidity, most of which count the number of incidents, for example, fractures avoided, tumours detected. In addition to such discrete outcome measures, there are continuous scales on which the severity of incidents can be depicted, for example, depression scales. The major deficiencies with the widely used clinical outcome measures are that firstly, they rarely account for duration, secondly, they use incommensurable outcome measures, and thirdly, rarely are preferences of the affected parties accounted for. Furthermore, these scales have their focus on the dimension(s) of health that the given treatment *intends* to impact upon. While negative 'side-effects' might sometimes be mentioned, they are not measured such that they can be compared in a meaningful way with the positive effects. There is also the issue of the unintended impact upon dimensions of health that are not being monitored.

This suggests that a useful health outcome measure for aiding resource allocation in health care should fulfil at least three requirements: (1) it should measure improvements in *both* mortality and morbidity; (2) it should use a generic (rather than a disease-specific) descriptive system for health so that comparisons can be made *across* programme areas; and (3) the valuation of the improvements should be based on the preferences of the affected parties. The *disability-adjusted life-year* (DALY) has been developed in order to calculate the loss, expressed in terms of years of life in full health, associated with premature mortality and morbidity, and is currently being used by the World Health Organization to calculate the 'global burden of disease' (Murray 1996). However, as it stands, the 22 health states used to calculate DALYs are based more on conditions than on generic health states and were valued by a panel of health care providers. For these reasons, we will focus our attention on the *quality-adjusted life-year* (QALY), which was designed specifically to meet the three requirements above.

7.3.2 Quality-adjusted life-years

A leading proponent of the QALY, Alan Williams, refers to the QALY algorithm as a 'sophisticated measure of health'. In general terms, there are three different *streams* of health. The first is a retrospective stream, looking at how many QALYs one has already had. The second is a prospective stream, looking at how many QALYs one can expect to have without an intervention. The third is also a prospective stream, but one which looks at how many extra QALYs one can expect to gain from an intervention. Since QALYs are developed for the purpose of comparing health *gains*, let us concentrate on this last stream.

For an individual, there are three possible dimensions of future health gain; improved health-related quality of life, a longer lifetime, and an increased probability of survival. A usual simplification is to subsume the probability parameter and refer to life expectancy. Quality of life (Q) is usually measured on a [0–1] scale where 1 refers to full health and 0 refers to death. Time (T) is counted in years. Consider now an intervention that improves longevity in full health by a given ΔT. The QALY gain (G) for this longer lifetime (T) is then:

$$\text{QALY}_{G-T} = Q * \Delta T = 1 * \Delta T = \Delta T. \tag{7.5}$$

Alternatively, consider an intervention that improves the health state by ΔQ, but does not change the longevity. The QALY gain for this improved

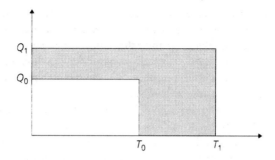

Fig. 7.1 The QALY model. The shaded area shows the health gains from treatment.

health related quality of life is:

$$QALY_{G-Q} = \Delta Q * T. \tag{7.6}$$

It follows from eqns 7.5 and 7.6 that a programme that improves mortality becomes *commensurable* in health outcome terms with one that improves morbidity.

However, many interventions improve both quality and length of life. Figure 7.1 illustrates the QALY gain by the shaded area, where we have assumed that the health-related quality of life remains constant—without treatment denoted as Q_0 and with treatment denoted as Q_1. Time is accordingly denoted T_0 without treatment and T_1 with treatment.

The general formula for a QALY gain can be written as:

$$QALY_G = Q_1 * T_1 - Q_0 * T_0. \tag{7.7}$$

where the first term on the right-hand side refers to the expected health with treatment and the second term refers to the 'no-treatment profile' (the formula assumes only those two outcomes but can be extended for any number of mutually exclusive events). This is all fine in theory, of course, but how in practice do we obtain reliable figures to be put into this general—and very simple—formula?

7.3.3 Measuring health-related quality of life

Length of life with and without treatment is normally obtained from mortality tables and survival rates, while the probability of successful outcomes might be given from operation mortality rates. The measurement of T enables comparisons on an interval scale, for example, the value of 10 years is twice as long as the value of 5 years (assuming there is no discounting, so that all years of life are given equal value, irrespective of when they occur— of which more below). Similarly, we need quality of life to be measured on a scale with similar interval properties.

There are three main methods that have been used to value Q—visual analogue scale (VAS), standard gamble (SG), and time trade-off (TTO). The VAS is a scale with fixed endpoints and equal intervals. It is usually illustrated vertically with a bottom value of 0, referred to as worst imaginable health (or dead), to a top of 100, referred to as best imaginable (or full) health. The respondent is then asked to locate a given description of a health state on this scale.

The SG presents a choice between being in a described health state for a given period of time for certain, and a risky option with one better and one worse outcome (usually full health and death). Respondents are then asked to specify the probability (p) of a successful outcome that would make them indifferent to being in the described health for certain, or go for the risky option. Formally, if Q_i is the value of the intermediate health state, p is the probability, Q_F is the value of full health, and Q_D is the value of death, then:

$$Q_i = p * Q_F + (1 - p)Q_D \rightarrow Q_i = p. \tag{7.8}$$

The left-hand side is the value of being in the described health and the right-hand side is the expected value of choosing the risky option. Hence, with $Q_F = 1$ and $Q_D = 0$, it follows that $Q_i = p$.

The TTO represents a choice between a longer life in an inferior health state and a shorter life in full health. Usually, respondents are asked to imagine themselves in the described health state for a period of T years (for example, $T = 10$), and then asked how many years they would be prepared to trade off in exchange for full health. Formally, if Q_i and Q_F are the described state and full health, t is the shorter time period in Q_F, and T is the given reference time, then:

$$Q_i * T = t * Q_F \rightarrow Q_i = t/T. \tag{7.9}$$

Many comparisons have been made of the health state values from these different approaches. The VAS tends to give the lowest values, and SG the highest, though not much higher than values from TTO. The theoretical reasons for these observed discrepancies appeal to intuitions. The VAS differs from SG and TTO in that it does not involve a choice that requires the respondent to give something up. When there is no sacrifice involved in giving a low value, it is easy to do so. With SG and TTO, a sacrifice *is* involved, either in terms of taking a risk of death (SG) or by giving up length of life (TTO). This would restrict one's propensity to state a low implied value. The major difference between SG and TTO is that of certainty in TTO versus *un*certainty in SG, so risk-averse respondents (that is, those who do not like taking risks) would give higher implicit health state values under SG. Also, in TTO, the fraction of time one is asked to trade off is that which lies at the end of a given time, and so if these distant years are given less weight (that is, if there is positive time preference), then respondents will give up these years more willingly.

In addition to these three methods for measuring an individual's value of Q, there is the person trade-off (PTO) method which looks at the social value of one health state compared to another (see Nord 1995). It does this by asking respondents to think about how many people would need to be treated in one health state to make it equivalent in social value terms to treating a different number of people in a different state.

Whatever valuation method is used, the use of commensurable outcome measures, such as the QALY, are primarily relevant for decisions about allocating resources *across* different programme areas, that is, in the determination of allocative efficiency. But whatever level we are making decisions at, we require information on costs.

7.4 Estimating costs—some key principles

7.4.1 Marginal costs

There is a saying that 'the only relevant costs are those from which you can escape'. These are the marginal costs, defined as the additional costs following a one-unit change in production. Marginal costs depend on *variable costs* only, which are costs that vary with the level of output. In addition to variable costs, there are *fixed costs*, which do not vary with the quantity produced. In practice, most decisions deal with the question of 'how much to produce' rather than 'whether to produce'. Therefore, the important information is the additional costs that follow an expansion, or the cost savings from a contraction. Before proceeding, some simple algebra may clarify. Total costs (*TC*) are fixed costs (*FC*) plus variable costs (*V*), the latter being a function of quantity, X:

$$TC = FC + V(X). \tag{7.10}$$

Average costs (AC) are simply total costs divided by the given quantity:

$$AC = TC/X. \tag{7.11}$$

Marginal costs (MC) are the extra costs of producing an additional unit. Since fixed costs by definition remain unchanged, only differences in variable costs matter:

$$MC = [FC + V(X+1)] - [FC + V(X)] = V(X+1) - V(X). \tag{7.12}$$

While marginal costs represent the information relevant to making a decision about whether to change the level of output, the types of cost information that most likely would be available in practice refer to average cost figures. It is much easier to obtain information on total costs and divide this by the given quantity produced than it is to make more detailed inquiries into exactly those resources required for making marginal changes in production.

Probably the most cited example of the practical importance of not relying on average cost estimates when determining the level of production is the study of the costs of guaiac stool testing (Neuhauser and Lewicki 1975). Based on the suggested guidelines by a group of medical specialists, six subsequent tests had been recommended for detecting cancer in the bowel. If performing all six tests, the average cost was estimated at US$2451 per detected cancer. However, because the incremental detection was strongly diminishing with additional tests, the marginal cost was US$47 million per detected case from performing the sixth test. While this extreme difference between marginal and average costs has been questioned, the important message from this example is that average cost figures are a misleading basis for determining cost consequences of marginal changes in an activity. This highlights the importance of information about marginal costs when making resource-allocation decisions.

7.4.2 Social costs

An economic evaluation is said to take the perspective of the wider society and not only a particular sector or institution within the society. This is a fundamentally different perspective from the type of financial appraisals usually done in private firms, where external effects on other actors are not included. Hence, a societal view implies that one would include the costs of resources used in any sector, not only a given hospital or a national health service. It would also include costs imposed on patients and their relatives.

In some textbooks one might find a distinction between three types of costs: direct costs (health care and other resources directly attributable to an intervention), indirect costs (what we have termed production losses), and intangible costs (the costs of grief and misery experienced by patients and their relatives). Direct costs are clearly the least controversial. Production losses represent a potentially big cost component, particularly for screening programmes that include large groups of people from the labour force, who lose productive time at work. Interestingly, the more productive a given group is, the more costly it is to screen them. The third type of costs is the most controversial to include. The grief and impediments due to an intervention is hard to quantify in monetary terms, and some of it may already have been taken account of in the health outcome assessments (as the difference between expected health outcome and current ill health).

Interestingly, the estimation of costs is often considered to be a more value-free venture than the estimation of health outcomes. But with costs, as with outcomes, analysts still have scope for manipulations. If the vested interest is one of making a new procedure look cheap, clearly the analyst could try to neglect those cost components that are not immediately visible. While trained economists surely hold different views on the relevance of including various cost components, they nevertheless agree that it is correct—as well as honest—to present a transparent costing assessment, that is, which items in which quantities at which unit values.

7.5 Discounting—a preference for the present

Adjusting for the different timing of costs and benefits is an essential feature of CBA and CEA. A discount rate is used as a 'time weight' to devalue the future—the stronger the preference for the present, the higher the 'time weight'. In health economic evaluations, the idea of discounting is controversial because it implies that future health gains are assigned lower social values than current health gains. An important question is whether health benefits should be discounted at a different rate than costs (that is, should we use a lower rate for health in the denominator than in the numerator of the CER?). An answer of 'no' is based on the 'eternal delay' implications of health investments. If the rate of decline of costs is greater than that for benefits, no programme would be undertaken within the current period because the cost per unit of benefit would always be less next period. However, this 'paralysing paradox' relates to budget allocation over time. If health planners have no scope for deferring current funds to future periods, but have to spend the current budget in order to achieve health policy objectives, then the idea of deferring all health care resources to the infinite future is irrelevant. Interestingly, the UK guidelines suggest a discount rate of 6% on costs, and 2.5% on health benefits.

7.5.1 The reasons for discounting

In the literature on discounting, two different reasons are given for applying a positive discount rate for public projects. First, there is the argument referred to as 'the social opportunity cost of capital', involving capital that would otherwise have been used in the private sector where it would have yielded a return. Thus, the rate of return on public projects should ideally be the same as the marginal private project that is being foregone. Second, because consumers have a preference for the present, they claim compensation for delaying consumption; the rate of this compensation is their *time preference rate*. Individuals' time preferences represent the aggregate of three distinct intertemporal concerns: the pure time preference, which refers solely to remoteness in time, and thus reflects their degree of impatience; the rate at which the marginal utility of increased future consumption diminishes; and uncertainty.

7.5.2 Some formulae and examples

The mathematical formulae are fairly simple as long as we operate with a constant discount rate, r, and discrete time. The present value of an item, Z, with a unitary value of 1, occurring at a given future time, t, is:

$$Z_{PVt} = \frac{1}{(1 + r)^t}. \tag{7.13}$$

It follows that the larger the discount rate and the further into the future we look, the higher the denominator becomes and, thus, the lower is the present value, Z_{PVt}. With this formula, we get the present value of a given number of health benefits that occur in a future time period, t.

If the benefits occur as a constant stream every year during the programme period, the present value of this stream is considered as an annuity. The formula for this annuity, A, with a unitary value of 1 (due at the end of each year) throughout the period, t is:

$$A = \frac{1}{(1 + r)} + \frac{1}{(1 + r)^2} + \frac{1}{(1 + r)^3} + \cdots + \frac{1}{(1 + r)^t}$$

$$= \frac{1 - (1 + r)^{-t}}{r} \tag{7.14}$$

Table 7.3 Some examples of the present values of a future event (Z_{PVt}) and a stream of events (A) depending on the discount rate (r) and time (t)

r (%)	Z_{PVt}		A	
	t = 5 years	t = 20 years	t = 5 years	t = 20 years
0	1	1	5	20
2	0.90	0.67	4.7	16.3
5	0.78	0.38	4.3	12.5
10	0.62	0.15	3.8	8.5

Table 7.3 shows the effects of different discount rates. A zero discount rate implies the same value to an event no matter how far into the future it occurs. A 10% rate could be used because it reflects time preferences for health (in fact, some empirical studies have found rates in excess of 10%). A rate of 5% has been the standard rate in applied economic evaluations of health care, and 2% comes close to the current UK recommendations for discounting health benefits.

So, the higher the rate, the less weight given to future gains. In addition, the choice of discount rate becomes more important for long-term programmes. If a 10% rate is used, a life saved in 20 years time is valued at only 0.15 of a life saved today. However, over a five-year horizon, these relative differences are much smaller: a life saved in five years is valued at 0.62 of one saved this year. Therefore, the health policy relevance of the discounting issue becomes more important for preventive programmes than for curative ones. When discounting over the course of an individual's *lifetime*, the annuity columns shows how life years are devalued, for example, using a 5% discount rate implies that 20 life years count for only 12.5 years in present value terms.

7.5.3 **Some views on discounting**

There are essentially three different normative views about how health should be discounted. The first is to use the same rate as for other goods in the economy. This argument emphasizes that capital allocated to health care has the same social opportunity cost as capital for other sectors. Accordingly, for consistency reasons, health gains should be subject to the same intertemporal criteria as other goods.

The second is to use a zero rate or one close to zero. Some medical ethicists hold that a life's value is the same no matter when it is saved and a QALY would similarly be equally valued whether it is gained this year or in the distant future. According to this moral principle, that all generations should be given equal weight (Parfit 1984), it follows that health gains be left undiscounted in economic evaluations.

The third view is that we should use the rate that best corresponds with people's preferences. This is the view held by economists with an affinity to the consumer sovereignty principle. However, many economists have been uneasy about individuals' impatience for own consumption; for example, Pigou (1932) suggested that 'our telescopic faculty is defective'. Following the argument by Sen (1982) that the individual—as a citizen—may have different time preferences for goods in a social context from those revealed in the context of private consumption, it might well be the case that the rate implied from an intertemporal choice between own health benefits differs from the rate implied from a societal intertemporal health choice.

These different normative views do not necessarily give different rates. For example, if people prefer that health gains should count equally no matter when they arise, the normative views (2 and 3) would give the same recommendation of a zero rate. There is, however, little (if any) empirical evidence for such preferences. Viewpoints 1 and 3 would give identical recommendations if the rate used for ordinary goods is based on people's time preferences, if people hold identical intertemporal preferences for health as they do for all other goods, and if these preferences are 'constant timing averse'. These requirements simply do not hold. There are theoretical reasons to believe that people have different time preferences for health compared to ordinary goods. Moreover, some studies suggest that people (and animals!) have *decreasing timing aversion* (that is, they attach less importance to a fixed time difference the farther into the future this difference is moved, Harvey 1994). As a consequence, so-called hyperbolic discounting models have been developed (see, for example, Cairns and van der Pol 1997).

Of these three different normative views, it is tempting to put a fairly rhetoric question: If we wish priority setting in health care to correspond with people's preferences, why should their intertemporal preferences not also count? A key issue in a societal judgement is how the present generation of citizens, with their current health care resources, would prioritize between the saving of lives now versus those in the future, and between improving the quality of lives now versus those in the future. The severe measurement problems inherent in the task of eliciting reliable rates represents a challenge both in terms of question format, as well as in choosing a context in which respondents are allowed sufficient time for deliberation and reflection.

Of particular relevance here is to come to terms with the reasons respondents give for assigning lower values to future health gains. From small convenience samples, we have indications that people expect technological progress will make it possible to provide future health gains at much lower costs. So, when respondents claim that more lives have to be saved in the future in order to forego some lives today, this reflects a view that these future lives could alternatively be saved at lower real costs in the future—a view that might be consistent with a preference for equal weight to lives saved in the future as lives saved this year. Clearly, more research is needed in order to understand whether the underlying reasons people state reflect something that can be explained by positive time preferences (that is, impatience, diminishing marginal utility, or uncertainty) or not.

Within a health context, the discount rate is sometimes perceived as an intertemporal *equity weight* that assigns relative social values to health gains depending on when they occur. Assuming constant technology over time, a discount rate of zero might be the most equitable, in that each generation counts the same. However, as opposed to such *inter*generational considerations, the impact of the discount rate leads to the opposite conclusion regarding *intra*generational equity (for a discussion, see Olsen 1994).

7.6 **Conclusion**

This chapter has sought to clarify key differences in the various types of economic evaluation techniques, and discussed normative issues related to the parameters that are included in the general economic evaluation formula (eqn 7.1).

First, the discount rate, r, has received much theoretical attention among health economists (including the two authors). At one end are those economists who take it as an exogenously given variable, determined by the treasury or the long-term interest rate. At the other are ethicists (and environmentalists) who are reluctant to its implications of devaluing the health of future generations. In yet other camps are health economists interested in preference elicitation and the scope for using the parameter as an equity weight. While we certainly find it a fascinating variable, it might seem that the theoretical interest it attracts does not necessarily correspond with its health policy importance, at least not for the majority of resources allocated to curative care.

Second, one costing issue deals with the inclusion of cost items outside the health service. Given the economic imperative that what matters are society's total resources required, not which sector or institution happens to carry the costs, this issue may seem a futile one. However, as noted throughout this book, publicly-funded health care resources are subject to different distributive criteria than are most other resources. Further, the opportunity costs of health care are health benefits foregone, while the opportunity costs of other resource uses might be anything, for example, lost leisure time, lost production of textbooks. It should perhaps not come as a surprise that non-economists question the extent to which such opportunity costs be included in a societal evaluation of health care.

Third, the most difficult parameters of them all are the quantification—and valuation—of the benefit items. When valued in money terms, interestingly, some evaluation techniques do not measure health *per se* but the impact that health changes have on the economy, be that cost savings or production gains. In that important respect, these techniques differ from the welfare economic cost–benefit analyses, which seek to value the benefits from health care based on individual preferences. Still, valuing health benefits in monetary terms involves measurement problems as well as controversial normative issues.

While we take a more optimistic view on measuring health benefits in health terms, these methodologies also have their measurement problems as well as normative issues. This is particularly so for the parameters which constitute the aggregated QALY. The probability term, for instance, can either be considered as a population based bio-statistical figure, or it can be considered an individual preference-based term that reflects risk attitudes. Some other QALY issues will be elaborated on in the next chapter.

In the economic evaluation literature there are controversies between advocates of the two different preference-based techniques—CBA versus CUA (see Table 7.1). The former have had a tendency to argue that CBA is 'theoretically correct' because it has foundations in new welfare economics. However, we believe this is not a positive issue, but a highly normative one. There is no such thing as a universally correct methodology for use in economic evaluations. Rather, the choice of approach crucially depends on the value judgement of the institution, whose decision making is being used in the analysis. Which method is 'right' depends on the answer to the questions in Table 7.4.

Table 7.4 CBA or CUA?

	CBA	**CUA**
What is the entity to be maximized?	Utility	Health
Who is to judge the goodness of the entity?	The affected consumer/patient	The affected patient, other members of society, or experts
How is the entity to be distributed?	Based on demands; willingness and ability to pay	Based on needs; expected health gains

CBA, cost–benefit analysis; CUA, cost–utility analysis.

This chapter has focused on the key parameters of an economic evaluation, and has tried to highlight some normative issues inherent in their assessments. The next chapter goes beyond these parameters and gives attention to ethical issues that lie outside what is normally considered to be the domain of economic evaluations.

Suggested reading

The standard reference is M. F. Drummond, B. O'Brien, G. L. Stoddart and G.W. Torrance (1997) *Methods for the economic evaluation of health care programmes 2ᵉ*. Oxford: Oxford University Press.

See also M. F. Drummond and A. McGuire (ed.) (2001) *Economic evaluation in health care: merging theory with practice*. Oxford: Oxford University Press.

The ethics of economic evaluation in priority setting

Economic evaluation techniques have been criticized for being too narrow, focusing on 'efficiency solutions' only and ignoring other priority-relevant considerations. This chapter considers additional issues related to equity and ethics, and how they might possibly be incorporated into a societal economic evaluation. Again, the rationale is to help in 'distributing health care'—but in an ethically preferred way.

Economic evaluation is unavoidably ethical in nature. Economists assume—as we will—that individual benefits are an important part of the social value of any health care programme. There then follows a number of important considerations when moving from individual benefits and towards social value. We are first faced with the question of how to aggregate individual benefits. Drawing largely on the work in Sections 3.2 and 3.3, the next section discusses how the benefits from economic evaluations can and should be aggregated.

There are then questions relating to the other things, besides individual benefit, that might be relevant to a decision at the social level which will not be relevant at the individual level (because it is assumed that any given individual would prefer more benefit to less). Some of these other things will relate to the other health characteristics of the potential recipients (Section 8.2) whilst others will relate to their personal characteristics—age, sex, and so on—more generally (Section 8.3).

The story in each of these sections suggests that all of the attributes relevant to a social decision can be incorporated into a single function to represent social welfare, that is, a social welfare function (SWF) that captures the relative weight given to each of the attributes. However, there are good reasons for supposing that this will not be possible. First, there are a range of measurement problems, some resulting from the fact that preferences are imprecise and partly constructed during the process of elicitation (Section 8.4). Second, in addition to the set of outcomes expressed in a SWF, there are a range of procedural and rights-based considerations which mean that not all the relevant attributes can be made commensurable with one another (Section 8.5). Despite these problems, however, using the results of economic evaluations is to be strongly preferred to *ad-hoc* decision making, and in the final section we discuss the merits of transparent and consistent decision making.

8.1 Aggregation issues

We saw in Section 3.2 that the conventional way in which benefits are aggregated in economics is by using the sum-ranking rule of the classical utilitarian philosophy. In this way, resources will be allocated so as to bring about the greatest overall benefit. There are, of course, other ways in which benefits can be aggregated, for example, by postulating a SWF that takes explicit account of the size of the population over which the benefits are distributed. And whether benefits are measured in monetary or health terms will determine what the maximand is.

8.1.1 Aggregation in monetary terms

We saw in Chapter 7 that gains and losses in cost–benefit analyses (CBA) are usually combined according to the potential Pareto improvement criterion, which simply means giving the same (unitary) weight to all gains and losses, irrespective of who receives them. However, a policy maker may wish to use a different set of distributional weights according to the prevailing distribution of income. The distribution of income matters because (1) an individual's willingness to pay (WTP) will be related to their *ability* to pay—rich people are able to pay more than poor people; and (2) the marginal utility that is sacrificed by (or gained from) a given monetary amount will be related to income—rich people lose (or gain) less in utility terms from a marginal change in their income (see the law of diminishing marginal utility in Section 2.2.1). For these reasons, a policy maker might wish to use distributional weights that give a relatively higher social value to gains and losses arising in lower income groups.

In addition, such weights might also be considered appropriate if there is some systematic relationship between income and the impact of the illness(es) in question. There is now a well-known association between social position and health, that is, poorer people tend to be sicker (see Section 1.4). In addition, the relative prevalence rates of different conditions might also differ across income groups. So, different relationships between income and certain illnesses will have different implications for aggregated WTP figures—not necessarily because the illnesses are considered to be of different severity, but simply because of differences in the income groups that the illnesses impact upon. Under such circumstances, policy makers would seem perfectly justified in using distributional weights to correct for this.

There is one other important, but very different, reason why a policy maker might not wish to aggregate gains and losses using unitary weights. This is because of the *identifiable victim effect*. This refers to the phenomenon that people are willing to spend greater resources on saving the life of an identified individual than on preventing a statistical fatality. Whether the effect is seen as an irrational bias or as a noble desire to aid others will owe much to the reasons that underlie it. Jenni and Loewenstein (1997) tested four possible explanations for the identifiable victim effect: (1) vividness (the fact that an individual can be visualized); (2) the certainty effect (the fact that one life can be saved for certain); (3) reference group size (a single individual is a reference group); and (4) *ex ante* versus *ex post* (which captures any residual effects). The size of the reference group was found to be the most significant effect. This means that distributional weights might also be used to take account of the relative fraction of the population affected by a particular intervention.

8.1.2 **The distribution of health benefits**

Although health benefits can be aggregated in any number of different ways, the sum-ranking (or maximization) rule forms the *de-facto* standard in 'cost–utility analysis' (CUA). The straightforward aggregation rule is then to take the average gain to the average individual and then multiply it by the number of people affected, N. For this algorithm to accurately represent the social value associated with health care interventions, all of the relevant parameters must have interval scale properties, that is, social value must be linear in N, besides the probability of success (p), quality of life (Q), and length of life (T). Linearity in N includes anonymity, because so long as there are N people in a particular health state at a given point in time, it does not matter who these people are.

However, there is now evidence that social value may not be linear in N, that is, people may strictly prefer a small benefit to the many, or even a large benefit to the few, even when overall benefits are the same. For example, Olsen (2000) found that a majority of respondents were not indifferent between two distributions with the same total gain. He suggests that there is a threshold level of benefits to the larger group above which people prefer to distribute gains to as many people as possible but below which they prefer to concentrate gains.

There is also evidence that people take account of how equally benefits are to be distributed across different groups when making prioritization decisions. For example, in a choice between two screening programmes, Ubel *et al.* (1996) found that half of respondents preferred the programme that could prevent fewer deaths but which could be offered to all citizens. However, in a follow-up study it was found that many fewer respondents held this preference when neither screening programme could be offered to everyone (Ubel *et al.* 2000). So, the evidence suggests a preference for the dispersion of benefits above a certain threshold, and a concentration of benefits below it. There would also seem to be a strong preference for providing everybody with a particular benefit.

8.2 The importance of different health streams

We have seen above that the size of health benefits matter, but so does the distribution of those benefits. In this section, we will consider other streams of health in addition to health benefits that might be relevant in determining the social value of a unit of additional health. In particular, we will look at the importance of the stream of health without treatment and the streams of health up to the point at which a decision is made. Let us begin with the stream of health without treatment.

8.2.1 The no-treatment health stream

Hadorn (1991) contends that people want to devote considerable resources to improving the health of seriously ill people, and in particular to those facing an immediate risk of death. He suggests that there is a conflict between cost-effectiveness and the 'rule of rescue' defined as the 'powerful human proclivity to rescue endangered life'. This means that the level of T without treatment would be weighted very highly and thus the value of life would then not be a linear function of the number of added years of life (over and above what would be suggested by discounting). Nord (1995) suggests that the no-treatment profile more generally (that is, the combination of Q and T) is important in its own right and argues that the social value of a given health gain is positively related to the initial severity of illness. The policy implication of this ethical viewpoint is that the quality-adjusted life-year (QALY) algorithm will give larger weights to those with poorer health prospects without treatment.

In general terms, and across a range of decision contexts, the empirical evidence suggests that people are willing to sacrifice gains in both length and quality of life in order to give priority to the most severely ill. There is also evidence akin to the threshold effect identified above. For example, Dolan and Cookson (2000) found that people were willing to make health gain trade-offs between patient groups once the differences in the number of life years gained went beyond a certain threshold. Furthermore, there is evidence that the *final* health state is also important, particularly in the context of a patient who cannot be returned to full health after treatment but whose health gain will be limited by disability (Dolan and Green 1998; Nord *et al.* 1999). In general, then, there is some empirical support for a *general rule of rescue*. In addition, *threshold effects* would appear to play an important part in the social value of gains in length and quality of life.

8.2.2 Age and the previous stream of health

The discussion so far has focused on what happens in the future. But it might also be ethically and policy relevant to consider previous streams of health. In other words, we might want to take account of how much health someone has accumulated in the past, as approximated by their age (but more accurately measured by the amount of QALYs they have enjoyed). There are three main concepts of 'ageism'. The first type of ageism is 'health-maximization ageism' (HMA) which is compatible with the assumption that each unit of health—expressed, for example, in terms of QALYs—is of equal value, irrespective of who receives those QALYs. *Ceteris paribus*, HMA will give priority to a younger person over an older one since the former will usually experience any health gains for longer.

The second type of ageism is 'productivity ageism' (PA). This gives priority to young adults because they are more productive at home and in society. The value given to a year of life at different ages will typically start at a relatively low value, increase rapidly to young adulthood, and then decrease more slowly towards old age. The age weights used in the calculation of the 'burden of disease' follow this pattern (Murray 1996).

The third type of ageism is 'fair innings ageism' (FIA). This looks at people's lifetime health, which could be quantified as the number of QALYs people can expect to have over their lifetime. Fair-innings ageism will give priority to a younger person over an older one because, *ceteris paribus*, the former has a smaller number of expected lifetime QALYs than the latter (Williams 1997). Fair-innings ageism will also give higher relative value to a person from a disadvantaged background than to a person from a more advantaged background, because, *ceteris paribus*, the former has fewer expected lifetime QALYs than the latter. Thus, HMA and PA both have a utilitarian basis, while FIA has an egalitarian basis.

There is empirical evidence to suggest that health gains to the young are weighted more highly than those to the old (Bowling 1996; Cropper *et al.* 1994; Lewis and Charny 1989). Whilst perceived differences in productivity across age groups alone are unlikely to explain the results in these studies, it is often difficult to tell how much of the preference for the young is due to the benefits to the young being greater (or being perceived to be greater) and how much is due to the young having lived for less time. Thus, it is difficult to distinguish between the different concepts of ageism from available empirical evidence.

Of course, age is merely a proxy for how much health someone has experienced and we would ideally like to know how many QALYs they have experienced up to the relevant decision point. And we might even like to know something more. In much the same way as it is possible to distinguish between QALYs gained as a result of *future* health care and those gained if no health care were provided, it is also possible to distinguish between QALYs gained as a result of *past* health care and those gained 'free' of health care (for a discussion, see Dolan and Olsen 2001).

8.3 **The importance of non-health characteristics**

The discussion above suggests that a person's *claims* to health care could be determined by characteristics of that person beyond their capacity to benefit, such as the severity of their no-treatment profile and their age. A claim is 'a duty owed to the candidate herself that she should have [the good]' (Broome 1991). Alternatively, as we saw in Section 5.4, claims could 'fall to the community to exercise duty over', and 'do not have to be recognized by the individual who has the claims' (Mooney 1998a). In what follows, claims refer to the extent to which a personal characteristic represents a *legitimate reason* for society to give a relatively higher or lower priority to a particular individual or group when distributing health care. Beyond the trade-off between 'need as capacity to benefit' (the QALY maximization argument) and 'need as ill health' (the rule of rescue argument), any additional claims depend on the *causes* of ill health and the wider *consequences* of an individual's improved health.

8.3.1 The causes of ill health

In discussing the importance of different health streams, we alluded to the potential relevance of where the responsibility of the need for health care lies. As Edgar *et al.* (1998) assert, 'It is possible to argue that [health] gains from treating ill-health which is brought about as a result of individual's own behaviour (smoking, drinking, engaging in dangerous sports, etc.) should be of lower value than those from treating ill-health for whom the victim was blameless.' This is obviously a controversial issue, both insofar as the degree of control that individuals have over their own actions is concerned, and the extent to which there exists a relationship between a particular action and subsequent ill health. We make no substantive claims about these issues. For our purposes, we need only to assume that all conditions can be located along an analytical spectrum from being *exogenously* determined (due to 'bad luck') through to being *endogenously* determined (as a result of well-informed 'own choices'). This distinction provides the reason why 'it is possible to argue' for giving different weight to the potential health benefits of different individuals or groups.

So far as the exogenous causes of ill health are concerned, some people may simply have been unlucky in the biological lottery to be born with an inherited disease, whilst others may have been the innocent victims of an identified cause of their ill health, for example, being hit by a car on the pavement. In such circumstances, where an individual experiences ill health through no fault of their own, it would seem that they have a relatively large claim to improved health through health care. With endogenous causes, ill health would rarely be entirely attributable to a person's own actions—even with smoking-related conditions, for example, there is much unexplained variation in who contracts the condition. Nevertheless, most people would consider ill health as a result of smoking to be located closer towards the endogenous end of the spectrum than ill health through genetic inheritance, and that is all that is required here is for smokers to be afforded a relatively smaller claim to improved health from health care than those with inherited diseases.

There is now empirical evidence that many people wish to give less priority to those who are considered to be in some way responsible for their ill health. For example, in two large-scale general population surveys, about half of the general public support discrimination against smokers (Bowling 1996; Jowell *et al.* 1996). However, using focus group discussions, Dolan *et al.* (1999) found that, whilst there was a majority view in favour of discriminating against those whose ill health is considered to be partly self-inflicted, this view provoked considerable discussion and dissent.

8.3.2 **The consequences of improved health**

Besides the individual benefit that a patient receives from treatment, there are also consequences *for other people*. These can be felt directly through a personal relationship or indirectly through economic effects. A distinction can then be made between the consequences for other peoples' *health*-related well-being and for their *wealth*-related well-being. The greater these consequences, the greater the claims to health care.

There is now strong evidence that people wish to discriminate in favour of those with dependants, particularly young children, but that they are less willing to do so on economic grounds (Dolan *et al.* 1999; Neuberger *et al.* 1998). These results could be explained by different degrees of *replaceability*. The effect that we each have on our families and friends cannot be easily replaced, but as breadwinners and taxpayers, most of us—much as we might like to think otherwise—are replaceable.

8.4 **Quantifying preferences**

The above discussion highlights that a composite measure of health benefits, expressed in monetary or health terms, is unlikely to pick up society's preferences over a range of attributes that have been shown to be relevant to resource-allocation decisions in health care. Proponents of economic evaluation have responded by arguing that preferences over these attributes could *in principle* be built into the benefits measure as weights, in order to derive a more complete measure of social benefits. This would allow us to specify a single SWF for use across a range of decision contexts. We will accept this principle in this section, and challenge it in the next section. We will concentrate here on how to elicit the kind of preferences that would be required to generate such an all-singing all-dancing SWF and then consider whether it is possible to do so *in practice*.

8.4.1 **The type of preferences required**

The measurement of preferences over the parameter values in a SWF raises a number of normative and methodological issues. We will focus here on one of the most important normative issues; namely, what *perspective* an individual should be asked to adopt. As discussed in Section 5.3, an individual might have a different set of preferences when asked to think of themselves as a consumer compared to a citizen. Therefore, the shoes they are placed in during a preference-elicitation study might have a significant effect on how they value the various arguments in the SWF.

Many economists would argue that a citizen's perspective that ignores self-interest represents an invalid means by which to determine priorities. If preferences that incorporate distributional considerations are required for informing allocation decisions, then economists usually recommend that the veil of ignorance be used—although often it is a much 'thinner' veil than that recommended by Rawls which denies the individual such things as the probability of emerging in a particular position in society (see Johannesson 1999). This operational device, which was introduced in Section 3.3, detaches the individual from their own vested interest by concealing their position in society, but still asks them to consider allocation decisions on the basis that they might ultimately affect them.

Unfortunately, the use of the veil of ignorance to determine a just distribution is hotly debated. Many philosophers are highly critical of the hypothetical nature of the contract that people are asked to enter into. For example, Dworkin (1977) questions whether such a contract is binding, arguing that 'the fact that a particular choice is in my interest at a particular time, under conditions of great uncertainty, is not a good argument for the fairness of enforcing that choice against me later under conditions of much greater knowledge'. The validity of hypothetical contracts is certainly questionable. Even if it were true that an individual would have consented to a particular distribution of resources before they knew what they needed, it does not necessarily follow that it would be fair to enforce that particular distribution on them when they know it is not in their actual interests.

The veil of ignorance has also been criticized on the ground that it links individual preferences from behind the veil with a just society once the veil has been lifted. Harris (1988) suggests that placing people behind a veil of ignorance does not ensure that the decisions that are made will be just. For example, people in the original position might choose a slave-owning society, gambling on emerging as a master rather than as a slave. Similarly, Barry (1989) argues that 'No adequate reason has ever been given . . . for identifying moral judgements with those made by someone trying to maximise his own prospects from behind a veil of ignorance.'

Others have been critical of the important effect that individual attitudes to risk behind the veil will have on society once the veil is lifted. Rawls' particular assertion that a 'rational egoist' would choose the maximin criterion from behind a veil of ignorance has been criticized and, although a veil of ignorance establishes impartiality, it is not enough to explain why people's preferences about gambles should provide any reason to favour one social situation rather than another. As Sen (1980) argues, 'It is far from obvious that prudential choice under as if uncertainty provides an adequate basis for moral judgement in unoriginal i.e. real-life positions.'

Although self-interest exists, it does not necessarily follow that it must be the basis for social welfare since society may adopt any objective or set of objectives that it desires. If an ethically defensible set of society-regarding preferences or social principles can be derived from forms of ethical reasoning that are clearly distinguished from mere self-interest—and, as Section 5.3 showed, we are not alone in thinking they can—then the citizen's perspective might well be a legitimate one.

Using people's preferences (either in their role as a consumer or a citizen) to estimate the parameter values in a SWF requires us, naturally enough, to quantify the relative value of all the arguments in that SWF. We now turn to consider whether it is possible to elicit this kind of information. In order to do so, we need to consider the nature of the preferences that are elicited to generate the weights for the various attributes that might go into a single SWF.

8.4.2 The nature of individual preferences

In standard economic models, it is simply assumed that each individual has an internally consistent set of preferences that will be *revealed* in market behaviour. Economists involved in eliciting *stated* preferences are clearly interested in the weights given to the various arguments in an individual's utility function, but they too have largely accepted the received wisdom, arguing that well-defined preference functions can be 'tapped into' by appropriate questions (see Fischhoff 1991). An implication of this view is that if a respondent gives different answers to two questions, then the questions must have been different. Therefore, economists involved in eliciting stated preferences tend to focus on ensuring that preference-elicitation questions are formulated and understood as intended, arguing that any 'slip' could invoke a precise, thoughtful answer to a 'wrong' question. Often a great deal of effort will go into the extensive piloting of questionnaires or survey instruments in order to ensure that the study is designed, so far as the researchers can tell, in ways that are most appropriate at generating meaningful answers to the intended questions.

However, the idea that people read their preferences off some in-built master utility function is called into question by psychologists and by the many studies which have shown that seemingly subtle changes in question framing or problem structure can change the stated preferences of respondents (see Slovic 1995). This evidence suggests that elicitation procedures can help to shape an individual's preferences. There seems to be increasing awareness of this and, as a result, many economists are attempting to gain a better understanding of the cognitive processes that a respondent uses in order to arrive at their responses. In this way, economists might become more able to understand any *biases* (resulting from framing effects and so on) that are present in their data.

However, many mainstream economists are yet to grasp the fact that their data may still be contaminated by *prejudices*, which are defined here as the difference between an individual's actual preferences (which might be racist, for example) and their preferences that have been suitably 'laundered' of those factors that are considered to be normatively unacceptable. Against this background, any study that does not provide a respondent with sufficient time to carefully consider their responses, as well as the opportunity to provide the (normatively acceptable) reasons underlying them, will not provide the *type* of stated preference data that we consider to be appropriate for informing resource-allocation decisions.

Whatever the precise details of future studies, the collection and analysis of qualitative data is crucial if we are to get a better understanding of individual preferences, and if the biases and prejudices inherent in them are to be reduced. Such procedures would of course be more expensive per response than postal surveys but would provide data that are more appropriate for use in policy making.

8.5 Quantifying rights and procedures

Even if it were possible to express all of society's preferences in a single measure, there are reasons why in principle a single all-encompassing SWF might not be the 'holy grail' that some economists apparently consider it to be. For example, using such a composite measure of consequences would mean that rights would be ignored (see Section 4.1). Within an outcome-focused SWF, one right is not considered to be morally superior to another. However, it is entirely possible (and perfectly consistent) for some rights to act as 'side-constraints' on public policy and so using QALYs does not mean that rights need to be ignored. But the important point in the context of this discussion is that the QALY, or some such outcome measure, is only operational once these constraints have been imposed.

In addition, using a composite measure of outcome would mean that any utility derived from procedures would be ignored. Section 3.4.2 showed that there are a range of justice rules—consistency, bias suppression, accuracy, correctability, representativeness, and ethicality—that may be relevant to how decisions are made. Insofar as these procedures involve opportunity costs in terms of outcomes or represent side-constraints on the maximand, a single SWF would not pick this up. However, it should be stressed that *any* measure of benefits does satisfy some of the procedural rules, such as consistency and transparency. And, in principle, it might be that some of the weights in the algorithm could relate to procedural aspects as well as to distributive considerations, although it remains to be seen whether this is possible or not.

Using a single SWF to inform resource-allocation decisions might also have important implications for the level of participation in the community. Because the welfare of the community might be an increasing function of the level of participation within it, there has been considerable interest in what the determinants of participation in society are (see McMillan and Chavis 1986; Oropesa 1992). However, remarkably little attention appears to have been paid to modelling participation as a function of the extent to which it is possible to influence decisions. This is surprising since participation is likely to be lower when individuals feel that they can have very little impact on decisions. For example, if there are explicit formulae by which health care resources are to be allocated within a community, there might be less incentive for individuals within that community to try to influence allocation decisions.

Of course, individual preferences may have been accounted for in the formulae and this will enhance their legitimacy. Moreover, people are likely to welcome the increased transparency in decision making that the formulae might bring about. However, no matter how deliberative the preference-elicitation procedure is, the incentive for direct public participation in the decision-making process would seem to be reduced once explicit formulae are generated. Because this in turn might undermine social solidarity, individuals might prefer for health care policy makers to have some discretion over the trade-offs they make so that participation can have a real impact on decisions at the margin.

Following these arguments, we think that the general public might prefer for only a limited number of attributes to be used as explicit criteria by policy makers, leaving the relative weight to be given to other attributes to be determined by context-specific participation. An additional reason for this public preference might be that people would like to understand the basis on which the algorithm is calculated, as well as to trust the validity of the numbers in the algorithm. The more criteria that individual benefits are weighted by, the more mystical it becomes, and thus, the less likely it is to be trusted. The simple QALY algorithm, for example, might be regarded as the most straightforward metric in the sense that it seeks to express only the individual benefits associated with alternative allocations. As a general rule, then, the fewer the parameters, the better.

All of this assumes, of course, that policy makers take into account the views of the public as expressed through participation. The political incentives that exist within most democracies suggest that policy makers cannot totally disregard these views. And presumably pressure groups and so on would not exist if they really had no impact on policy. It also assumes that participation, through increased social solidarity, is welfare enhancing. But, naturally, the fact that participation in the form of pressure groups, lobbying , and so on has the potential to affect policy means that there are incentives for rent-seeking behaviour on the parts of groups and organizations. However, it remains that providing some incentives for participation might result in higher social welfare than providing no incentives at all.

8.6 **Conclusion**

In this chapter, we have shown that there is much more to social welfare than simply individual benefits—and much more to social welfare than simply the unweighted aggregation of those benefits. Interestingly, it seems to us that health economists have been much more willing to accept that 'a $ is a $ is a $' than that 'a QALY is a QALY is a QALY'. The monetary metric of CBA is much more acceptable to mainstream economists than the health measures of CUA, and so it would seem that if you insist on benefits being measured in monetary terms, then you are more willing to accept an aggregation rule that is based on potential Pareto improvements (notwithstanding some attempts to estimate distributive weights based on a diminishing marginal utility of income).

This is interesting but not without reason. If you accept 'a $ is a $ is a $', then you can close your eyes to the normative problems that assuming anything else raises. Of course, giving all dollars equal weight is a normative judgement in itself, but it just *appears* to be less like one (not least because it takes the prevailing income distribution as given and, hence, optimal). And weighting all dollars equally avoids all the practical problems associated with trying to elicit weights—it is simply so much easier to give everyone the same weight. But once you commit the heresy of abandoning a monetary measure of benefits in favour of a health-related one, then you might as well go the whole hog and chuck out simple aggregation rules too.

In fact, you might as well chuck out the whole idea that there exists a social welfare maximand at all.

Hang on a minute! As economists, we would not—could not—go that far. It may not be possible to express all the things that we value about the public provision of health care in a single SWF, but this should not stop us from trying to quantify the quantifiable. It should not stop us from eliciting preferences—yes, even imprecise ones—about the various trade-offs that people would be willing to make between the various more readily quantified arguments in the SWF. It should not stop us from taking that information and using it as a basis (rather than as a rigid rule) for resource-allocation decisions in health care. And it should not stop us from seeking to elicit preferences about the contexts in which other less quantifiable arguments in the SWF might matter.

Suggested reading

See Nord, E. (1999) *Cost-value analysis in health care: making sense out of QALYs.* Cambridge: Cambridge University Press.

Mooney, G. (1998) 'Communitarian claims' as an ethical basis for allocating health care resources. *Social Science and Medicine*, 47, 1171–80.

Williams, A. (1997) Intergenerational equity: an exploration of the fair innings argument. *Health Economics*, 6, 117–32.

Towards a new health economics?

This final chapter draws out some of the implications from each of the preceding chapters for the future of health economics, as it is applied to the issue of distributing health care.

This chapter is loosely organized around the preceding eight chapters of the book. But rather than summarizing these chapters, we aim to provide material which enables us to suggest future directions for health economists. This agenda is largely driven by our own interests in the issue of how health care should be distributed in publicly funded health care systems, but, even in this sub-set of health economics, our suggestions are far from being exhaustive—they simply represent our own views about where priority should lie, and readers are of course free to disagree with us. We begin by looking at where the boundaries of health economics lie.

9.1 The boundaries of health economics

The two-by-two table in Fig. 9.1 focuses on inputs (resources) and outputs (impacts on people). In relation to inputs, a health economic analysis might concentrate on health care resources only or it might include all those resources that are required for the desired outputs. The outputs of the programme can be defined according to its impact on health or utility. Health is a narrower entity than utility—and narrower than definitions of individual well-being. There is, however, no real consensus about precisely how broad or narrow the definition of health should be (see the different dimensions used in the health state descriptive systems reported in Table 1.1).

One other, and perhaps more important, distinction can be made between health and utility. Whilst utility is a highly subjective thing, health (and well-being for that matter) can be valued by someone other than the individual experiencing it. Most economists are familiar with the concept of subjective utility, and might consider the focus on health to be much more controversial, particularly if it is the preferences of other people (such

Outputs / Inputs	Health	Utility
Health care	1	2
All resources	3	4

Fig. 9.1 The domain of health economics.

as the general population) who determine the value of their possible states of health. But, as we discussed in Section 3.1, in the case of distributing health care, what matters might not be an individual's subjective assessment of their own utility from health care but rather society's valuation of the improved health that health care may produce.

Health care is clearly a sub-set of all the resources that impact upon health (or well-being or utility). It is fair to say that health economics, as an applied sub-discipline, would be more accurately described as health *care* economics (boxes 1 and 2 in Fig. 9.1). It has taken the health care system as its starting point and applied the tools of economics to it. The health care system in the USA is more market oriented than in Europe and comes closer to 'conventional economics', and so there is more attention paid to box 2. However, the focus of attention of most health care systems in which there is considerable willingness to contribute towards the health care of others is usually on health, that is box 1.

In fact, it will usually be the case that we demand health care *for ourselves* because it contributes towards our health—the demand for health care is derived from the demand for health. Therefore, health economists have traditionally—and we suggest correctly—focused on health rather than utility. This implies that there is something special about health compared to some other arguments (like going on holiday) in an individual's utility function.

It has been recognized for a long time that there are many things that contribute towards health besides health care. There is an ever-expanding literature on the determinants of health that health economists are increasingly contributing towards, that is, analysis in box 3. The final box in Fig. 9.1, box 4, is concerned with the allocation of resources insofar as they contribute towards utility. Whilst within the core of welfare economics, such general considerations would normally be seen as being outside of health economics.

We suggest, therefore, that health economics is concerned with the three shaded boxes, 1–3. The vertical choice between box 1 and box 2 depends on the objectives of the health care system. The horizontal choice is a tricky one. Economists would generally subscribe to the view that 'a cost is a cost is a cost' no matter who bears it, and this is consistent with what we have learnt about including all societal costs in an economic evaluation. The problem is that the opportunity costs in terms of foregone health are different when considering health care costs compared to the costs borne by other institutions or individuals. The alternative to spending health care resources to improve A's health is to spend those resources on improving B's health. However, the foregone benefits of the additional costs of A's treatment are unlikely to be B's health—if the additional costs of A's treatment were their lost earnings, then the foregone benefits of A's treatment would be their private consumption. Given that the opportunity costs of these other resources are not necessarily measured in terms of foregone health, we would welcome more research on the distributive implications (for health) of accounting for the additional cost items.

9.2 The demand for curves

Many non-economists appear to perceive economics as 'all about demand and supply'. So, it might come as a shock to them to find out that there is a debate within health economics about whether the demand curve for health even exists (there was a plenary session at the 1999 International Health Economists Association Conference entitled 'Should the demand curve be abolished?'). The demand curve (Fig. 9.2) is intended to illustrate a demand function in which the quantity demanded (Q_D) is a function of price (P) alone, *ceteris paribus* (everything else held constant), that is, $Q_D = f(p, \ldots)$.

This curve tells us how many units of a good a consumer will purchase at different prices. For most goods most of the time, the demand curve is assumed to slope downward from left to right, that is, demand falls as price rises, and vice versa. In a market, if there is limited availability of services, the price of those services will be set high enough to ensure that there is no excess demand for them.

So, what's the problem then? Well, there are at least two. The first is that most health care markets do not ration by price. Whether and when you get a particular treatment does not turn on your answer to the question

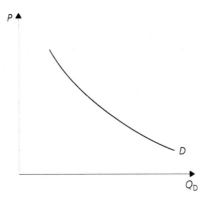

Fig. 9.2 The demand curve.

'What are you willing to pay for it?' but on someone else's answer to the question 'How much do they need it?' This leads us into the second problem; namely, that there are many things which influence the observed utilization of health care in addition to price (without wishing to be patronizing, stop and think for a moment about what influences your own decisions about whether to consume health care and at what levels—this might make you wonder why health economists have focused on 'price–quantity' demand curves when 'other things–quantity' demand curves might be much more useful).

Consider the following sequence of events: *demand → need → utilization.* According to the economic theory discussed in Chapters 2 and 4, *demand* reflects the autonomous choices of well-informed consumers. The closest we get to witness this is when someone visits their doctor. During this consultation there is, by definition, an interaction between 'the demander' and 'the supplier' in which the better-informed supplier recommends health care that they think the demander will *need*. Depending on the extent to which the patient takes the doctor's advice, *utilization* of health care is then observed (we are not regarding the consultation itself as utilization here). Hence, the observed utilization of health care depends on the preferences of the consumer *and* on the recommendations of the supplier.

There is a danger in focusing on the demand curve in that it may easily lead analysts, and policy makers, to use the price mechanism to solve problems of 'excess demand'. Thereby, all other factors that influence doctors' recommendations, and thus influence the utilization of health care, are forgotten about. Once we recognize that there is strong interaction between the demand and supply sides, that patients do not make consumption decisions in a vacuum, and that suppliers might even induce demand for their services, then we require types of analyses that lie outside of neo-classical economics and which recognize the interdependencies between demand and supply.

9.3 **Justice and fairness: societal judgements**

Amartya Sen has suggested that economics has two different origins; the 'engineering' approach, which is concerned with logistic issues, and the 'ethics' approach, which encompasses political philosophy. Sen has argued that economists have increasingly pursued the former approach at the expense of the latter. This certainly could help explain why economists have focused on supposedly technical considerations of efficiency rather than on issues of justice and fairness. But health economists cannot hope to address issues of how to distribute health care without considering the ethical principles upon which distribution is to be based. An efficient and equitable distribution of health care requires us to devote much time to defining and understanding precisely what these concepts mean.

Health economics—like many other sub-disciplines in economics—has been largely based on utilitarianism. This means that the preferred distribution of health care is the one that maximizes the sum total of gains. The focus on health—so long as we seek to maximize it—has still to be seen as lying broadly within the utilitarian tradition. A number of health economists are now arguing that other points on the utility possibility frontier (UPF) might be preferred to the maximizing one, and some are even beginning to elicit the preferences of the general public about such issues as the nature and the extent of the trade-off between maximizing health and reducing inequalities in health.

Still, and this is important to most economists, an optimal distribution is required to be located *on* the UPF—any point inside it represents waste. We believe that the reason for the lack of understanding of interior points is the consequentialist nature of economics. Health economists might contribute more towards the debate about how to distribute health care if they gained a better understanding of the role and relevance of rights and procedural justice, as well as knowledge of the code of medical ethics. As intimated at in Chapter 3, it is a real challenge to try and distinguish interior points that have an explanation and justification in theories of procedural justice and medical ethics from those that represent mere waste.

9.4 **The market fails—but so may the government**

So much of health economics has been about how the market for health care differs from other markets. Kenneth Arrow's article (1963) is seen by many as being the beginning of health economics, and in it he considers uncertainty and the role of insurance. The market can certainly fail due to such things as asymmetric information about the distribution of risk in a given population. To mitigate such problems in the financing of health care, governments around the world have stepped in to make the market work better and many countries have even replaced the market with 'public health care'.

Irrespective of the extent to which a goverment allows the market to allocate health care, governments and non-market forces still play a big part in influencing the behaviour of suppliers of health care. In most countries we observe quite strict regulations of providers in terms of professional codes of conduct and clinical guidelines. It might be fair to say that some health economists have got a bit obsessed with the idea of supplier-induced demand, but the powerful position of doctors in most health care systems means that markets cannot be relied upon to provide sufficient checks on their behaviour.

But like most drugs, there may be unintended side-effects—just as markets fail, governments can fail too. Private markets, which will fail to internalize any externalities, might not produce the type and level of health care that society wants. Public health care systems might work such that 'the public gets what the public wants'—but they might do so inefficiently and at high cost. It has long been argued that the public sector is less efficient than the private sector because, in the absence of market forces, managers in the public sector have greater discretionary power than those in the private sector and are thus freer to pursue their own objectives. Indeed, a whole sub-discipline of economics called 'public choice' has developed to look at precisely this issue.

Once the ethical framework has been established and the objectives of the health system have been set, it is really an empirical question about whether the market or the state gets us closer to where we want to be relative to how much it costs us to get there. But this question, like so many, gets hijacked by ideology and political dogma.

9.5 **Caring for others**

There are many reasons why we care about the health of other people. Some of these are selfishly motivated—their health affects our health or wealth. But other reasons are motivated by altruism or simply because we care. If it is the health of other people that we care about (rather than their access to, or use of, health care), then we will be more willing to pay—to put our altruistic money where our mouths are—for health care that has the greatest impact on health. And if we care about the health of some people (such as the poorest or sickest members of society) more than others, then we will be more willing to cross-subsidize the health care of those who can afford it least or who will be worse off (in wealth or health terms) without it.

Our concern for the health or well-being (rather than the utility) of others suggests that we are *paternalistic altruists* rather than general altruists—we wish people well, not happy. In this way, society's preferences legitimize the focus of health economists on health rather than on utility. But it does, once again, raise the question of 'What is health?' It also leads us to consider—in ways that health economists have not really done so thus far—what types of public health care would gain the greatest public support. We suspect that we feel obliged to subsidize health care (or health *cure*) for which there are very few close substitutes—a patient with a brain tumour, for example, cannot really be given much else so we feel obliged to pay for their treatment. With health *prevention*, however, there are 'many ways to skin a cat' and we may feel under less obligation to buy someone health care when they can alternatively 'buy' themselves a healthier lifestyle that would yield the same risk reduction.

Interestingly though, recent debates in the UK and elsewhere about whether and how to ration such things as the drug viagra for erectile dysfunction suggests that the distinction between health and well-being is very blurred. It could be that the answer to the question of why health care is so special lies as much in the *causes* of losses in well-being as in the *consequences* of health care. In other words, health care might be special because people care about losses that are the result of more 'health-related' causes. In a time when more and more 'lifestyle drugs' become available, it will become increasingly important for health economists to contribute to the debate about what should and what should not be provided by publicly funded health care systems.

9.6 **Purchasing and providing health care**

Although details differ between countries, all health care systems have mechanisms designed to control costs. Once society has determined the slice of tax or social insurance revenues devoted to its public health service, the third-party payer must ensure that expenditures do not exceed the budgets so allocated. Many health care systems are characterized by monopoly or near monopoly in raising revenues and in allocating resources so as to have some control of the revenue–expenditure identity. But, of course, systems of private insurance funding face the same identity—an insurance company cannot reimburse more expenditures than it can cover by the revenues generated from the sale of its insurance contracts.

While there are efficiency arguments for publicly funded health care, where the premiums are linked to incomes, we have emphasized that the choice of financing system is also a highly normative one. Publicly funded health care follows from an objective of 'from each according to ability, to each according to need'. Furthermore, we have argued that public finance does not imply public provision. A range of different reimbursement systems exist between purchasers and providers, all of which can be judged according to cost containment (keeping expenditures in line with revenues) and efficiency (fulfilling societal objectives for the distribution of health care).

To meet these objectives, many health care systems (like the National Health Service in the UK) have introduced competition between suppliers in the form of internal markets or the purchaser–provider split. The idea is that monopoly power on the purchasing side and competition on the providing side will strengthen the hand of payers relative to suppliers, and will act as a force for cost control. However, this requires that hospitals are provided with the appropriate incentives to maximize the objectives of purchasers and that those on the demand side (government, purchasing agencies, and general practitioner fundholders) have sufficient information about performance to monitor suppliers. These issues are certainly important topics in health economics, although they have been discussed extensively in this book, which focuses on distributing—rather than financing—health care.

9.7 Economic evaluation

Evaluations seek to provide information that helps policy makers make decisions about what they do with the resources at their disposal. Until recently, evaluations in health care were solely clinical, investigating the efficacy (can a product work?) and effectiveness (does it work?) of an intervention. Economic evaluation investigates efficiency: Is this the most cost-effective alternative, creating the greatest benefit per unit of cost? Encouragingly for economists, there has been an increased emphasis on cost-effectiveness in many countries. In the UK, for example, the National

Institute for Clinical Excellence has been established to consider the reimbursement of new technologies and the results of economic evalaution studies are crucial in determining this.

The economic evaluation of health care programmes has two main features: to value both the inputs (costs) and outputs (consequences) of any activity and to compare two or more alternatives (one of which may be to do nothing at all). Economic evaluation is seen by some doctors as an exercise in cost cutting and is regarded by others as unethical. Of course, much depends on which ethical basis is being referred to, but we cannot identify a major conflict between medical ethics (see Section 3.4.3) and economic evaluation since dealing fairly with patients ultimately involves considering opportunity costs.

The two main forms of economic evaluation are cost–benefit analysis (CBA), where benefits are measured in monetary units, and cost–effectiveness analysis (CEA), where benefits are expressed in a single measure, such as life years gained or quality-adjusted life-years (QALYs). Some economists have tried to build a welfare economic bridge between the two forms of analysis. However, rather than attempting to find a bridge that is able to reconcile the central conflict between utility and health maximization, we suggest that attention is instead focused on the debate about the appropriateness of CBA *vis-à-vis* CEA.

Whilst this debate is taking place, those involved in economic evaluations should, so far as possible, undertake evaluations that facilitate cross-study comparisons. Too often the results from one economic evaluation cannot be compared with those from another and thus very little information is provided to help macro-level decision making. It is of course difficult to standardize analyses when there is so much disagreement about what constitutes 'best practice' but, in CEA, for example, there is now general agreement that the health state descriptive system should be generic, that the valuation method should be preference based, and that the source of values should be a representative sample of the general population.

9.8 Beyond health benefits

Cost-effectiveness analyses are concerned with the maximization of health benefits and, as such, ignore (or, more accurately, are neutral towards) distributional concerns. But there are many things besides health benefits that might be considered relevant when distributing health care. Many of these relate to the *claims* that an individual has on resources. For example, those whose health will be worse without treatment, those who cannot be considered to be responsible for their illness, those with family commitments, or those with rare skills may all have a greater claim to beneficial health care than others.

Health economists have been much more willing to accept that 'a $ is a $ is a $' in CBA than they have been willing to accept that 'a QALY is a QALY is a QALY' in CEA, but it is important that consideration be given to how to weight benefits under both forms of analyses. Some health economists have been active in developing methodologies that allow for a range of different equity concerns to be incorporated into the social welfare calculus. However, even if it were possible to express all of these equity concerns in a single measure (and there are many methodological reasons to suppose not), there are reasons why *in principle* this all-singing all-dancing measure might not be the Holy Grail that many economists apparently consider it to be.

For a start procedural utility is ignored and it is hard to see how this could be made commensurable with distributive principles. An equity-weighted measure of benefits might also have important implications for the level of participation in the community, in that the use of explicit formulae to allocate health care resources might mean that there is less incentive for individuals within that community to try to influence allocation decisions (this could also be seen as a good thing of course).

Our own proposal would be to identify those equity considerations that the general public consider to be relevant, look at the reasons why they consider them to be relevant, and then look broadly (but not precisely) at the relative importance attached to them. We contend that health economists involved in preference-elicitation studies cannot at some level avoid inquiry into the *reasons* for responses. Therefore, future research efforts should be directed towards (1) setting out the normative criteria by which to judge the reasonableness (or otherwise) of reasons for responses; and (2) qualitative research methods to provide evidence about the reasons behind responses.

9.9 **A new normative health economics?**

This book has focused on some of the important normative issues involved in discussions about how to distribute health care. However, we have been unable to provide definitive answers to the economic and ethical questions surrounding health care rationing because the answers depend on the value judgements that are made.

Economists will often begin by adopting the value judgements of welfarism—that individuals are the best judges of their own welfare and that social welfare is represented by some aggregation of the preferences of sovereign consumers. But the rationale behind many public health care systems is very different—individuals are not always the best judges of their own welfare so far as the consumption of health care is concerned and the social value of health care is much more than the aggregation of patient-centred benefits. Health economists who wish to have a real effect on health policy either need to persuade those involved in distributing health care to adopt their paradigm or they need to adopt the paradigm adopted by their health care system. Whilst many health economists are wedded to the traditions of welfare economics, it would seem that many others are more pragmatic and begin by considering which paradigm is best suited to the objectives of the system.

It seems to us that the ideas of 'non-welfarism' in health have emerged as a result of searching for a normative rationale for public health care. A key distinction between the 'welfarist' and 'non-welfarist' approaches—as we interpret them—is whether individuals can have preferences as citizens that exist independently or beyond their preferences as consumers. In other words, do the utilities of consumers or patients *ex post* differ from the values of citizens or tax payers *ex ante*? We believe that more research should be undertaken into eliciting preferences for alternative distributive principles. If citizens preferred health care to be distributed according to the principle 'to each according to need' rather than 'to each according to willingness (and ability) to pay', welfarists would have a hard job convincing the public that the latter principle is still theoretically correct. But economists more generally could sleep a little more easily at night, safe in the knowledge that their health care system was satisfying the preferences of the population—the societal preferences of citizens, rather than the individual preferences of consumers, that's all.

References

Chapter 1 **Health care and health**

Brazier, J. E., Deverill, M., and Green, C. (1999) A review of the use of health status measures in economic evaluation. *Journal of Health Services Research and Policy*, 4, 174–84.

Evans, R. G. and Wolfson, A. D. (1980) Faith, hope and charity: health care in the utility function. Discussion Paper. Department of Economics, University of British Columbia, Vancouver.

Evans, R. G., Barer, M., and Marmor, T. (ed.) (1994) *Why are some people healthy and others not? The determinants of health of populations.* New York: Gruyter.

Richardson, J., Hawthorne, G., and Day, N. A. (2001) A comparison of the assessment of quality of life (AQoL) with four other generic utility instruments. *Annals of Medicine*, 33, 358–70.

WHO, http://www.who.int/whosis/

Chapter 3 **Justice and fairness**

Broome, J. (1991) *Weighing goods*. Oxford: Basil Blackwell.

Culyer, A. J. (1990) Commodities, characteristics of commodities, characteristics of people, utilities and the quality of life. In *The quality of life: perspectives and policies* (ed. S. Baldwin), pp. 9–27. London: Routledge.

Daniels, N. (1985) *Just health care*. Cambridge: Cambridge University Press.

Elster, J. (1992) *Local justice: how institutions allocate scarce goods and necessary burdens*. New York: Russel Sage.

Habermas, J. (1984) *The theory of communicative action* (two volumes translated by T. McCarthy). Boston: Beacon Press.

Harsanyi, J. (1955) Cardinal welfare, individualistic ethics and interpersonal comparisons of utility. *Journal of Political Economy*, 63, 309–21.

Kant, I. (1785) *Fundamental principles of metaphysics of ethics*, English trans. by T. K. Abbott. London, Longmans (1907).

Levanthal, G. S. (1980) What should be done with equity theory: new approaches to the study of fairness in social relations. Chapter 2, in *Social exchange: advances in theory and research* (ed. K. Gergen, M. Greenberg, and R. Willis). New York: Plenum Press.

Nozick, R. (1974) *Anarchy, state and utopia*. New York: Basic Books.

Rawls, J. (1971) *A theory of justice*. Cambridge, MA: Harvard University Press.

Rawls, J. (1982) Social unity and primary goods. In *Utilitarianism and beyond* (ed. A. Sen and B. Williams), pp. 159–85. Cambridge: Cambridge University Press.

Sen, A. (1987) *On ethics and economics*. Oxford: Basil Blackwell.

Sen, A. and Williams, B. (1982) Introduction. In *Utilitarianism and beyond* (ed. A. Sen and B. Williams), pp. 1–21. Cambridge: Cambridge University Press.

Chapter 4 **Efficiency-motivated responses to market failures**

Clark, D. and Olsen, J. A. (1994) Agency in health care with an endogenous budget constraint. *Journal of Health Economics*, 13, 231–51.

Culyer, A. J. (1989) The normative economics of health care finance and provision. *Oxford Review of Economic Policy*, 5, 34–58.

Evans, R. G. (1984) *Strained mercy: the economics of Canadian health care*. Toronto: Butterworths.

Folland, S., Goodman, A. C., and Stano, S. (1997) *The Economics of health and health care*. London: Prentice Hall.

Fuchs, V. (1986) Physician induced demand: a parable. *Journal of Health Economics*, 5, 367.

Grossmann, M. (1972) On the concept of health capital and the demand for health. *Journal of Political Economy*, 80, 223–55.

Hurley, J. (2000) An overview of the normative economics of the health sector. In *Handbook of health economics* (ed. A. J. Culyer and J. P. Newhouse). Amsterdam: Elsevier.

Krasnik, A., Groenewegen, P. P., Pedersen, P. A., von Schatten, P., Mooney, G., Goltschan, A., Flierman, H. A., and Damsgaard, M. T. (1990) Changing remuneration systems: effects on activity in general practice. *British Medical Journal*, 330, 1698–701.

Williams, A. (1988) Ethics and efficiency in the provision of health care. In *Philosophy and medical welfare* (ed. J. M. Bell and S. Mendus). Cambridge: Cambridge University Press.

Chapter 5 **Equity-motivated responses to market failures**

Barr, N. (1993) *The economics of the welfare state*. London: Weidenfeld and Nicolson.

Broome, J. (1991) *Weighing goods*. Oxford: Basil Blackwell.

Culyer, A. J. (1989) The normative economics of health care finance and provision. *Oxford Review of Economic Policy*, 5, 34–58.

Etzioni, A. (1986) The case for a multiple utility conception. *Economics and Philosophy*, 2, 159–83.

Harsanyi, J. (1955) Cardinal welfare, individualistic ethics and interpersonal comparisons of utility. *Journal of Political Economy*, 63, 309–21.

Mooney, G. (1998) 'Communitarian claims' as an ethical basis for allocating health care resources. *Social Science and Medicine*, 47, 1171–80.

Rousseau, J. J. (1762) *The Social Contract*. (1998 translation). London: Wordsworth.

Sen, A. (1987) *On ethics and economics*. Oxford: Basil Blackwell.

Chapter 6 **Providing health care: finance and regulation**

Evans, R. G. (1997) Going for the gold, the redistributive agenda behind market-based health care reforms. *Journal of Health Politics, Policy and Law*, 22, 427–65.

Chapter 7 **Economic evaluation techniques**

Beattie, J., Covey, J., Dolan, P., Hopkins, L., Jones-Lee, M., Loomes, G. *et al.* (1998) On the contingent valuation of safety and the safety of contingent valuation: part 1—caveat investigator. *Journal of Risk and Uncertainty*, 17, 5–25.

Cairns, J. A and van der Pol, M. M. (1997) Constant and decreasing timing aversion *Social Science and Medicine*, 45, 1653–9.

Harvey, C. M. (1994) The reasonableness of non-constant discounting. *Journal of Public Economics*, 53, 31–51.

Koopmanschap, M. A., Rutten, F. F. H., van Ineveld, B. M., and van Roijen, L. (1995) The friction cost method for measuring indirect costs of disease. *Journal of Health Economics*, 14, 171–89.

Murray, C. J. L. (1996) Rethinking DALYs. In *The global burden of disease* (ed. C. J. L. Murray *et al.*). Harvard: Harvard University Press.

Neuhauser, D. and Lewicki, A. M. (1975) What do we gain from the sixth stool guiac? *New England Journal of Medicine*, 293, 226–8.

Nord, E. (1995) The person-trade-off approach to valuing health care programmes *Medical Decision Making*, 15, 201–8.

Olsen, J. A. (1994) Persons vs years: two ways of eliciting implicit weights. *Health Economics*, 3, 39–46.

Olsen, J. A., and Richardson, J. (1999) Production gains from health care: what should be included in cost-effectiveness analyses? *Social Science and Medicine*, 49, 17–26.

Olsen, J. A., Donaldson, C., and Shackley, P. (2001) *Sensitivity of 'willingness to pay' relative to theoretical construct: a review of the results from EuroWill*. Presented at the World Conference on Health Economics, York.

Parfit, D. (1984) *Reasons and persons*. Clarendon Press: Oxford.

Pigou, A. C. (1932) *The economics of welfare* (4th edn). London: Macmillan.

Sen, A. (1982) Approaches to the choice of discount rates for social benefit–cost analysis. In *Discounting for time and risk in energy policy* (ed. R. Lind). Baltimore: Johns Hopkins University Press.

Tengs, T. O, Adams, M. E, Pliskin, J. S., Safran, D. G., Siegel, J. E., Weinstein, M. C., and Graham, J. D. (1995) Five hundred life-saving interventions and their cost-effectiveness. *Risk Analysis*, 15, 369–90.

Torrance, G. W. (1986) Measurement of health state utilities for economics appraisal. *Journal of Health Economics*, 5, 1–30.

Weinstein, M. C., Siegel, J. E., Garber, A. M., Lipscombe, J., Luce, B. R., Manning, W. G. *et al.* (1997) Productivity costs, time costs and health-related quality of life: a response to the Erasmus Group. *Health Economics*, 6, 505–10.

Chapter 8 **The ethics of economic evaluation in priority setting**

Barry, B. (1989) *Theories of justice*. Hemel Hempsteaf: Harvester Wheatsheaf.

Bowling, A. (1996) Health care rationing: the public's debate. *British Medical Journal*, 312, 670–4.

Broome, J. (1991) *Weighing goods*. Oxford: Basil Blackwell.

Cropper, M. L., Aydede, S. K., and Portney, P. R. (1994) Preferences for life saving programs—how the public discounts time and age. *Journal of Risk and Uncertainty*, 8, 243–65.

Dolan, P. and Cookson, R. (2000) A qualitative study of the extent to which health gain matters when choosing between groups of patients. *Health Policy*, 51, 19–30.

Dolan, P. and Green, C. (1998) Using the person trade-off approach to examine differences between individual and social values. *Health Economics*, 7, 307–12.

Dolan, P. and Olsen, J. A. (2001) Equity in health, the importance of different health streams. *Journal of Health Economics*, 20, 823–34.

Dolan, P., Cookson, R., and Ferguson, B. (1999) Effect of discussion and deliberation on the public's views of priority setting in health care: focus group study. *British Medical Journal*, 318, 916–19.

Dworkin, R. (1977) *Taking rights seriously*. Cambridge: Cambridge University Press.

Edgar, A., Salek, S., Shickle, D., and Cohen, D. (1998) The ethical QALY: ethical issues in healthcare resource allocation. Haslemere, UK: Euromed Communications.

Fischhoff, B. (1991) Value elicitation, is there anything there? *American Psychologist* 46, 835–47.

Hadorn, D. C. (1991) Setting health-care priorities in Oregon—cost-effectiveness meets the rule of rescue. *Journal of the American Medical Association*, 265, 2218–25.

Harris, J. (1988) *More and better justice*. In *Philosophy and medical welfare* (eds. M. Bell and S. Mendus). Cambridge: Cambridge University Press.

Jenni, K. E. and Loewenstein, G. (1997) Explaining the 'identifiable victim effect'. *Journal of Risk and Uncertainty*, 14, 235–57.

Johannesson, M. (1999) On aggregating QALYs: A comment on Dolan. *Journal of Health Economics*, 18, 381–6.

Jowell, R. J. *et al.* (ed.) (1996) British social attitudes. The 13th report, Aldershot: Dartmouth (for) Social and Community Planning Research.

Lewis, P. A. and Charny, M. (1989) Which of 2 individuals do you treat when only their ages are different and you cant treat both? *Journal of Medical Ethics*, 15, 28–32.

McMillan, D. and Chavis, D. (1986) Sense of community, a definition and theory. *Journal of Community Psychology*, 14, 6–23.

Mooney, G. (1998a) 'Communitarian claims' as an ethical basis for allocating health care resources. *Social Science and Medicine*, 47, 1171–80.

Mooney, G. (1998b) Beyond health outcomes: the benefits of health care. *Health Care Analysis*, 6, 99–105.

Murray, C. J. L. (1996) Rethinking DALYs. In *The global burden of disease* (eds. C. J. L. Murray and A. D. Lopez). Harvard: Harvard University Press.

Neuberger, J., Adams, D., MacMaster, P., Maidment, A., and Speed, M. (1998) Assessing priorities for allocation of donor liver grafts, survey of public and clinicians. *British Medical Journal*, 317, 172–5.

Nord, E. (1995) The person-trade-off approach to valuing health-care programs. *Medical Decision Making*, 15, 201–8.

Nord, E., Pinto, J. L., Richardson, J., Menzel, P., and Ubel, P. (1999) Incorporating societal concerns for fairness in numerical valuations of health programmes. *Health Economics*, 8, 25–39.

Olsen, J. A. (2000) A note on eliciting distributive preferences for health. *Journal of Health Economics*, 19, 541–50.

Oropesa, R. (1992) Social structure, social solidarity and involvement in neighborhood improvement associations. *Sociological Inquiry*, 62, 107–18.

Sen, A. (1980) *Choice, welfare and measurement*. Oxford: Basil Blackwell.

Slovic, P. (1995) The construction of preferences. *American Psychologist* 50, 364–71.

Ubel, P. A., Dekay, M. L., Baron, J., and Asch, D. A. (1996) Cost-effectiveness analysis in a setting of budget constraints—is it equitable? *New England Journal of Medicine*, 334, 1174–7.

Ubel, P. A., Baron, J., Nash, B., and Asch, D. A. (2000) Are preferences for equity over efficiency in health care allocation 'all or nothing'? *Medical Care*, 38, 366–73.

Williams, A. (1997) Intergenerational equity: an exploration of the 'fair innings' argument. *Health Economics*, 6, 117–32.

Chapter 9 **Towards a new health economics?**

Arrow, K. (1963) Uncertainty and the welfare economics of medical care. *American Economic Review*, 53, 941–73.

Index